Evidence-based Wound Management

by

MAUREEN BENBOW BA, MSc, RGN, HERC

University College, Chester

W
WHURR PUBLISHERS
LONDON AND PHILADELPHIA

© 2005 Whurr Publishers Ltd
First published 2005
by Whurr Publishers Ltd
19b Compton Terrace
London N1 2UN England and
325 Chestnut Street, Philadelphia PA 19106 USA

British Library Cataloguing in Publication Data

A catalogue record for this book
is available from the British Library.

ISBN 1 86156 474 0

Typeset by Adrian McLaughlin, a@microguides.net
Printed and bound in the UK by Henry Ling Limited at the Dorset Press.

Contents

Preface

Wound management has become a highly specialized field of nursing over the past 15 years, causing much confusion for practitioners who, in the past, have viewed it as simple 'dressing changes'. The aim of this book is to assist students of health care positively to appreciate the complexity of this vast and growing subject, so that they benefit from a clear presentation of current knowledge and become confident enough to apply their new knowledge in practice. Wound management and the preservation of skin and tissue integrity affect all patient groups, nursing specialties and care settings.

Only the increasing number of technologies and therapies available to practitioners matches the challenge of increasing numbers of chronic and acute wounds as the population ages. This is an exciting time for specialists, wound care researchers and practitioners who manage wounds, to work together to bring about the best outcomes for patients.

By working through the contents of the book the reader will develop an understanding of the origins of wound management and how modern wound technology has evolved.

Experience as a ward manager, educator and specialist nurse has rewarded me with the skills and knowledge to recognize and appreciate the difficulties that present in practice. It is hoped that, by providing a comprehensive, step-by-step learning resource, the difficulties will become challenges and problems will be solved more easily.

In summary, this book aims to provide the student of health care with a basic set of tools for starting to experience and enjoy the provision of high-quality wound management.

Maureen Benbow

Introduction

This book has been written as a continuing, comprehensive resource for the student of nursing and its allied professions. Up-to-date knowledge is presented concisely with references to the sources of literature on which the theories and principles underpinning practice recommendations are based.

The reader is led along a pathway from the origins of ancient wound management and how they link with the modern technological advances and beyond, towards propositions for the future. Reference to wound management research is presented in relation to the level of evidence that is currently acknowledged by the experts.

The emphasis throughout the book is on conservative approaches to direct wound management with active general support of the patient, i.e. the correction of underlying and influencing factors, infection control and improvement of the medical and nutritional condition.

The basic principles of wound management relate to what can be done to provide the optimal microenvironment for repair, one that encourages rather than impedes healing, based on research evidence. The wound-healing process is explained with the evolution of treatments and therapies discussed in more depth in the subsequent chapters.

Recommendations are supported by guidance from the Department of Health, the National Institute for Clinical Excellence and the University of York systematic reviews, with findings incorporated into the text. Each chapter follows the same format. The relevant information is supplemented with interesting facts, followed by student exercises at the end of each chapter.

Real-life patient experiences are described, used to illustrate various points and emphasize the patient-centred approach to wound management. A comprehensive glossary of terms helps to explain the confusing and often complicated terminology, and is provided to complement the text.

The final chapters concentrate on managing patients with wounds and exploring opportunities for providing high-quality care, the possible environments of care, roles of key personnel, education and where research is taking wound management in the future.

Acknowledgement

The author and the publishers thank **Coloplast Ltd** and **Smith and Nephew Healthcare Ltd** for their contributions towards the cost of producing the colour plates in this book.

CHAPTER ONE

Wound care: past beliefs and practices

Doctors, nurses, hospitals and dressings are not recently discovered entities; they have all been around for many thousands of years in various forms. The first doctors lived about 4000 years ago in Egypt and before that time there were witch doctors and healers. The documented history of wound management dates back to 2000 years BC (Gelbart 1999) and the need for cleanliness in relation to wounds is mentioned as early as the fifth century BC. Humans have developed the propensity to survive, repair damage and fight off invaders. Healing and the immune responses, it is now known, are natural processes and are inextricably linked.

In the past, well-meaning individuals, lacking modern-day knowledge, tried to assist the body in this natural process of repair by sometimes making erroneous and appalling judgements.

It was not until the nineteenth century that the prevailing ignorance began to disperse and be replaced by logical theories based on important scientific discoveries relating to how wounds heal. Key discoveries relate to the identification of the factors that retard the rate of healing and what can be done to alleviate or minimize them. Currently knowledge, skills and resources are available to provide the optimal rate of healing but work is ongoing to explore ways in which the actual rate of healing can be positively influenced in all groups of patients with wounds.

From myths, beliefs, fallacies, witchcraft and mysteries

Early wound management comprised what would now be considered an outrageous array of natural substances used to cleanse, cover, treat, aid suppuration, staunch bleeding and prevent infection. In the early days, wounds were usually sustained through accidents involving animals, other people and rudimentary tools. Today injuries are more complex, involving faster, mechanical devices that impart more severe tissue damage.

1

Wound management, in turn, has developed into a complex science moving away from covering wounds with leaves, birds' feathers, sphagnum moss, cobwebs, animal dung, meat, the heads of soldier ants, boiled puppies and leather to covering them with hydrocolloids and foams, from irrigating wounds with wine, sea water, phenol and oil to irrigation with warmed sterile saline, and from the use of figs to de-slough necrotic wounds and sodium hypochlorites to hydrogels and sterile larval therapy (Westaby 1985).

Westaby (1985) believes covering the wound with leaves, birds' feathers and leather to be an instinctive method used not only to stem bleeding, but also to cover the wound from sight. There appears to have been an illogical urge to exclude air from wounds through the ages which has unknowingly protected injured tissue from bacterial infection. Milk and human urine have been used in the battlefield to cleanse wounds in the absence of sterile cleansing fluid. Honey has been favoured for thousands of years because it was relatively pathogen free and provided a bland covering to the wound; currently it is enjoying a revival in popularity.

However, as long ago as the time of Hippocrates (460–370 BC) caution and cleanliness in wound care were promoted: clean wounds were to be left without a dressing and others to be washed and covered with clean linen soaked in wine or vinegar (Hauben 1985).

'Laudable pus'

The removal of dead or devitalized tissue has moved in and out of fashion over the ages. Hippocrates advocated the 'scarification' of ulcers, but later in the Middle Ages 'laudable pus' became the trend and followers of this concept believed that it was a prerequisite to wound healing. In the pre-scientific era, it was thought that the production of pus in a wound was an essential part of healing and that, if it did not appear, the physician must induce it. This was achieved by placing certain noxious substances on the wound which often resulted in sepsis, gangrene and death. This was the concept of 'laudable pus' that underpinned medical observation at the time: pus formed in most wounds and, in patients in whom pus did not appear, death followed. What the physicians did not realize was that death was caused by failure or inability of the immune response to cope. Thus, it was assumed that the production of pus was a prerequisite to healing. Pasteur and Lister (Lawrence 1994) later refuted the theory of 'laudable pus' with the discovery of micro-organisms and their role in the infective disease process.

Débridement

One theory supporting the removal of necrotic tissue is that 'nature' hates a space and the necrotic tissue that occupies the space prevents healing. However, convention dictates that the presence of necrotic tissue in a wound impedes the progress of the important first stage of healing – the inflammatory phase – and should be removed so that healing may progress. The other important factor to be considered when a wound is filled with necrotic tissue is the risk of infection. Necrotic tissue is almost always colonized with bacteria and failure to remove it may result in clinical infection (Thomas 1990).

The conventional treatment for cavity wounds pre-1943 was packing with Vaseline gauze and immobilization; however, during World War II Italian doctors proposed a new method. Contrary to tradition, they wanted to cleanse and débride the wounds, which resulted in improved healing. The origins of this method were actually traced back to the thirteenth century but demonstrated how entrenched practitioners may become (Popp 1995).

The primary closure of wounds with a form of suture dates back to Egyptian times, although closing wounds was not favoured because of the high risk of infection. A thorn was used as the needle with a thread attached to it for suturing wounds; later the Greeks and Romans used needles with eyes made of bronze, copper or iron (Leaper 2000). By the late fifteenth century, it was realized that suppuration (the production of pus) was unnecessary for wound healing and wound edges were apposed using bandage. The use of tourniquets and pressure to arrest bleeding has prevailed for thousands of years with cobwebs used as a haemostat (Leaper 2000).

A short history of wound cleansing

Effective wound cleansing is essential to avoid infection and allow healing at the optimum rate. Different wound-cleansing solutions have been advocated to disinfect wounds and reduce the spread of bacteria. Hypochlorite solutions have been around since 1820, used to prevent the spread of puerperal sepsis (Thomas 1990). These solutions were used to bleach and disinfect utensils as well as wounds. They were originally introduced for the treatment of infected wounds before the discovery of antibiotics and antiseptic agents. As the result of a chemical reaction between the solution and body proteins, hypochlorite solutions were thought to be able to break down necrotic tissue, pus and plasma; however, it was necessary to use large volumes of solution. Barton and Barton (1981) found that the use of hypochlorites could cause the release of endotoxins and other toxic material from bacteria in the wound, resulting in acute oliguric renal failure. Hydrogen peroxide solution has been used for its mechanical detergent action resulting from the release of oxygen gas. It has limited antibacterial properties because it is deactivated by body proteins. There is a possibility that, if used under pressure or in closed body cavities, oxygen bubbles may pass into the bloodstream and cause an air embolus (Sleigh and Linter 1985). Proflavine cream has only a mildly bacteriostatic action against Gram-positive bacteria as a result of its inability to be released from the cream (Thomas 1990).

Cetrimide has an antibacterial action against Gram-positive and Gram-negative bacteria and has been used to cleanse dirty and infected wounds. It is not recommended for routine use in non-infected wounds because even in low concentrations it has cytotoxic and cytostatic properties (Thomas 1990). Chlorhexidine is a detergent that is effective against a wide range of bacteria and is useful for the first aid of dirty, contaminated, traumatic wounds, but not as a routine cleansing agent.

The antiseptic, povidone–iodine, has been popular for its broad spectrum of activity but, similar to other antiseptic solutions, its activity is reduced in the presence of pus and exudate. Various enzymatic preparations have been used to de-slough necrotic wounds for which evidence has emerged suggesting that they are no more effective than modern-day hydrogels.

Over recent years, there has been a move away from the harsh cleansing solutions to use of physiological or 0.9% saline for the routine cleansing of wounds as a result of the detrimental effect on healing tissues of hypochlorites and antiseptics. Disruption of capillary circulation in granulation tissue, increased inflammatory response, retarded collagen formation, cytotoxic properties and weakened scar tissue are valid reasons why such solutions should be avoided for routine wound cleansing. Sterile 0.9% saline is the safest solution to use, because there is no evidence that antiseptics reduce the bacterial count in a wound. With much traditional nursing mystique attached to the 'non-touch, aseptic technique', 'clean hand–dirty hand' and very specific methods of wound cleansing, confusion abounded. These methods persisted for many years, incorporating the use of dressings that were traumatic to healing wounds and unacceptable to patients, because of their odour and trauma on removal, but also, paradoxically, to fulfil the practical assessment criteria demanded in nurse training.

The method of wound cleansing also came under scrutiny with questions about whether the traditional swabbing with cotton-wool balls or gauze was appropriate. It is now generally accepted that, when a wound needs to be cleansed, gentle irrigation with warmed 0.9% saline or water is preferable to avoid the shedding of cotton fibres into the wound, which can act as a focus for infection (Draper 1985). Wounds need cleansing only when they are heavily contaminated with particles of dirt or other organic material, or contain excess exudate or old dressing material (Miller and Dyson 1996, Lawrence 1997). As to the method, common sense should dictate basic principles such as how to avoid contaminating the wound by thorough hand washing and appropriate handling of dressings.

Moving into the present day

Major change occurred during the late nineteenth century when Lister demonstrated the importance of good aseptic practice in medicine and surgery, which also had a significant influence on the way wounds were managed. Lint, gauze and cotton dressings replaced the former non-sterile dressings. Absorbent padding (Gamgee Tissue), sometimes impregnated with iodine or phenol, was developed followed by the introduction of 'tulle gras'-type gauze dressings impregnated with paraffin. The first 'tulle gras' dressing was produced by Lumiere during World War I from an open-weave cloth impregnated with soft paraffin containing 1.25% Balsam of Peru (mild antiseptic). Many of the 'tulle gras' dressings were prepared from net curtain before impregnation with soft paraffin, packing and sterilization (Thomas 1990). These products are available today consisting of bleached cotton, or cotton and viscose gauze, and a reduced load of soft paraffin to reduce their occlusive properties and risk of maceration. Tulle dressings were manufactured as carriers for a range of medications: local anaesthetic agents, sulphonamides, antibiotics, vitamins and honey. The use of medicated tulle dressings declined when the risk of antibiotic resistance was identified and patients were found to develop sensitivity reactions to the materials.

Major change occurred in the latter part of the twentieth century with the transformation of simple dressings to the more complex wound management products and materials. This change was stimulated by the research conducted by Winter (1962), who discovered that a wound in a domestic pig healed more quickly under an occlusive material than under a dry dressing. The principle of moist wound healing was defined and established to influence the future of modern wound management significantly.

Following this discovery, further research was undertaken to develop and produce a whole new generation of products that would optimally support the healing process. The introduction of semi-permeable film dressings, hydrocolloid dressings, foam dressings, hydrogels and more have revolutionized the way wounds are managed today. The discovery of antibiotics and the explosive expansion of knowledge about wound management have largely replaced the need for natural non-sterile 'dressings' and the suppuration of wounds, thought to be necessary for healing for hundreds of years.

Exudate

Excessive exudate production can present major problems to both the patient, in terms of soiling clothes and bed linen, and the nurse who must devise methods for controlling it through frequent dressing changes. Current research is focusing on the positive features of exudate, which include its active antibacterial properties and the fact that it is rich in nutrients. Analyses of the components of exudate from acute wounds are being compared with that from chronic wounds. This is to ascertain what differences there are in its composition, which may provide insight into the development of products or devices that can transform the slow healing of a chronic wound into the healing of an acute wound. However, the problems relating to the management of excess wound exudate, while retaining moisture at the wound surface, remain.

The focus on chronic wounds

As knowledge of wound healing and management developed, it concentrated mainly on acute traumatic and surgically induced wounds until the need to address the management of chronic wounds was realized (Watret and White 2001). Previously, wound management had been the responsibility of doctors, then medical students, and eventually ward sisters and now nurses. Consequently, much of the research and innovation over recent years have been in relation to the treatment of chronic wounds, which have generally become the domain and responsibility of nurses. Currently, living in a cost-effective society that demands proof of efficacy and value for money in health care, it is difficult, in spite of the many significant advances, to demonstrate evidence-based practice. Newer therapies abound and are quickly accepted as custom and practice with little evidence available to support their use. The search for evidence continues to underpin the basic principles of wound care and inform best clinical practice.

Student exercises

• Explore the rationale for the use of hypochlorite solutions in wound care.
• Examine the properties of traditional dressings such as gauze and Gamgee, and compare them with modern-day dressings such as hydrocolloids.

CHAPTER TWO
Cells, tissues and skin

The integumentary system

The complex integumentary system comprises skin, hair, nails and various multicellular exocrine glands. The skin is the largest and most visible organ system of the body, so that when something goes wrong it is immediately apparent. Visible signs of other system dysfunction can be identified through changes in skin colour or sensitivity, e.g. flushed skin indicates pyrexia. The integument or skin weighs approximately 3 kg and covers about 1.7 m² (Bevan 1978). About one-third of the total circulating blood volume is contained in the skin (Herlihy and Maebius 2000). Skin is able to withstand a number of mechanical and chemical assaults and is capable of self-regeneration (Wysocki 2000). The thickness of skin varies from 0.05 mm in the tympanic membrane to 6 mm in the soles of the feet (Wysocki 2000).

Skin comprises two distinct layers: the outer or surface layer called the epidermis and the inner layer, the dermis, which is anchored to the subcutaneous layer (Herlihy and Maebius 2000). Each layer of skin is described in detail.

The structure and function of skin (Figure 2.1)

The outer layer of skin or epidermis consists of superficial, stratified, squamous epithelial cells or keratinocytes; it is avascular and waterproof. Oxygen and nutrients, however, diffuse into the lower dermis from the underlying dermis. The five layers of the epidermis comprise: the outer stratum corneum, stratum lucidum, stratum granulosum, stratum spinosum and stratum germinativum or basal layer. The stratum corneum is composed of dead keratinized cells, which are abraded daily when a person washes, scratches or exercises (Wysocki 2000). The human epidermis is renewed every 1530 days depending on the area of the body, age and other

7

factors (Junqueira et al. 1977). Keratin is an insoluble protein also found in the hair and nails which is resistant to changes in pH, temperature and chemical digestion by trypsin and pepsin (Tortora and Anagnostakos 1987). Keratin is capable of absorbing large quantities of water, which may lead to maceration (a softening or sogginess of the tissue owing to retention of excessive moisture (Cutting 1996)) and skin breakdown (Lloyd and Moody 1999).

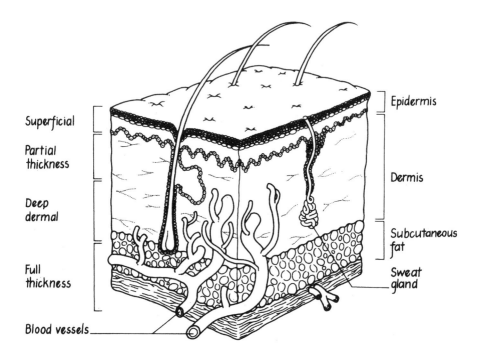

Figure 2.1 The structure of the skin (from Bosworth Bousfield C, 2003, with permission).

The second layer of epidermis, the stratum lucidum, varies in thickness – it can be as little as one to five cells thick and is found where the epidermis is thicker, such as in the soles of the feet (Wysocki 2000). The stratum granulosum is one to three cells thick and contains flattened and irregularly shaped cells. It is at this level of the epidermis that the keratinocytes become non-viable. The stratum spinosum or prickly layer contains keratinocytes that are polyhedral in shape and differentiate from the basal cells below (Lookingbill and Marks 1993).

The stratum germinativum, or basal layer, consists of mitotically active basal keratinocytes which can be regarded as the 'stem cells' of the epidermis (Lookingbill and Marks 1993). This layer contains rête ridges to anchor the epidermis and melanocytes (cells that synthesize melanin to give skin its colour). Sunlight stimulates increased production of melanocytes. Genetic differences control the number of pigment cells that are incorporated into the epidermis and therefore how dark the skin becomes. The absence of a pigment-forming enzyme in the skin causes albinism (Herlihy and Maebius 2000). Any breach in the skin extending to this level exposes the body to infection. Cells in the stratum corneum are constantly sloughing off and being replaced by other cells moving up from the deeper layers (Herlihy and Maebius 2000).

The basal membrane zone or dermoepidermal junction separates the epidermis from the dermis and contains fibronectin and collagen. The dermis, also called the 'true skin' (Herlihy and Maebius 2000), is the thickest skin layer (2–5 mm) composed of dense fibrous connective tissue and contains numerous collagenous and elastic fibres (Tortora and Anagnostakos 1987, Wysocki 2000) surrounded by a gel-like substance. This structure makes the dermis strong and stretchable. If the skin is overstretched, however, the dermis may be damaged and form pink lines that gradually turn white, known as 'stretch marks' (Herlihy and Maebius 2000).

The capillary network lies directly under the basement membrane to supply oxygen and nutrients to the overlying epidermal cells (Tong 1999). Collagen is the body's main structural protein and, in the skin, is secreted as tropocollagen (Wysocki 2000). This is the protein that gives skin its tensile strength and acts as a buffer to external pressure. Elastin provides the property of elastic recoil to the skin (Wysocki 2000). Also found in the integument are accessory structures such as hair follicles, sebaceous glands, sweat glands, nervous tissue and some muscle tissue. Many of the nerves have endings called sensory receptors that detect pain, temperature, pressure and touch (Martini and Bartholomew 2000).

Approximately 3 million eccrine sweat glands in the skin produce water, waste salts and urea. There are different types of eccrine glands, e.g. in the ear, which produce wax and in the genital and axillary areas where the apocrine glands produce a thicker fluid that skin bacteria break down to produce body odour. Sebaceous glands adjacent to hair follicles produce sebum to oil the hair and lubricate the skin by keeping sweat on the epidermis (Herlihy and Maebius 2000). Macrophages and fibroblasts, key cells for healing, are found in the gelatinous fluid matrix of the dermis. Pacinian corpuscles in the dermis are the nerve endings responsible for detecting pressure and direct the brain to initiate movement by reflex action when a person becomes uncomfortable (Martini and Bartholomew 2000).

The hypodermis or subcutaneous layer lies beneath the dermis comprising adipose tissue and connective tissue that attaches the skin to deeper structures such as muscles and bones plus a network of blood vessels (Wysocki 2000). Major functions of the layer of 'fat' cells are to protect infants and small children from injury (Bridel 1993), to insulate from cold and to provide an energy reserve. The distribution of fat changes as people mature so that, in men, fat accumulates around the neck, upper arms, lower back and buttocks whereas in women fat accumulates in the breasts, buttocks, hips and thighs. Both males and females may accumulate excessive amounts in the abdomen (Herlihy and Maebius 2000).

The many important functions of skin are closely interlinked to its structure as the largest body organ.

Protective function

The outer layer of skin covers and protects underlying tissues from trauma, chemicals, water, ultraviolet radiation (melanin) and infection (via the skin immune system and secretions from the sebaceous glands), and prevents loss of body fluids and electrolytes to maintain homoeostasis (Wysocki 2000).

Human skin in healthy adults is inhospitable to pathogenic organisms (Parker 2000). There are many harmless bacteria and fungi inhabiting the skin and it is not until the opportunity arises for penetrating the skin that they become pathogenic. If the skin is breached and the bacteria are transferred to another area of the body, cellulitis (a diffuse inflammation of connective tissue) or wound infection may occur (Parker 2000). Skin has two main lines of defence: the horny keratin layer that acts as a physical barrier when intact and the bactericidal skin secretions and resident flora. The protective function of skin is key to preventing or ameliorating many dry skin conditions such as some types of eczema, contact dermatitis and psoriasis, which cause dry, cracking skin that allows ingress of irritants and allergens (Lookingbill and Marks 1993).

The Langerhans' cells, tissue macrophages, which ingest and digest bacteria and other substances, an antigen-presenting cell found in the epidermis and mast cells, which contain histamine, comprise the skin immune system (Tortora and Anagnostakos 1987). Melanocytes produce melanin which is the pigment that darkens skin and when exposed to sunlight secretion increases (the summer tan) in an attempt to protect deeper layers of tissue from ultraviolet light. Freckles and moles are examples of melanin that becomes concentrated in local areas (Herlihy and Maebius 2000).

Maintenance of body temperature

Skin regulates heat loss to the environment through the thermoregulatory mechanisms of sweating and vasoconstriction/vasodilatation. Most heat (80%) is lost centrally. Body temperature is usually maintained at

approximately 98.6°F or 37°C by the hypothalamus – the body's thermo-
stat. When there is deviation from the normal, three structures in the skin
assist in temperature regulation: the blood vessels, the sweat glands and
the arrector pili muscles (Herlihy and Maebius 2000).

The normal functioning of these structures allows more blood to flow to
the skin surface transferring heat from the deeper tissues. Sweat glands are
stimulated to produce sweat for evaporation, which aids cooling. In an
attempt to retain body heat the opposite effects of vascular constriction,
inactivity of sweat glands, activation of peripheral nerves and contraction
of the arrector pili muscles ('gooseflesh') occur, causing an increase in the
production of heat.

Heat can be lost or dissipated through radiation, conduction, convection and evaporation (Table 2.1). Heat is lost through radiation when the
heat from a warm body is lost to the cooler air of a cold room; it is lost by
conduction when a warm body is in contact with a cold surface, e.g. the use
of a cooling blanket to reduce very high temperatures in clinical practice.
Heat is lost by convection or the loss of heat by air currents, e.g. using a fan
to cool a patient and evaporation when liquid becomes a gas. The latter
happens when alcohol is rubbed on the skin: it evaporates and cools the
skin. In conditions of extreme humidity sweat cannot evaporate from the
surface of the skin so the body does not cool by evaporation and radiation;
however, it will still be able to cool by convection and conduction (Herlihy
and Maebius 2000).

Table 2.1 Heat loss regulation by the skin

Temperature below normal	Temperature above normal
Reduced peripheral circulation Vasoconstriction Reduced direct heat loss from blood Reduced water evaporation through skin	Increased peripheral circulation Vasodilatation Increased direct heat loss from blood Increased water evaporation through skin
Sweat glands do not produce water for evaporation	Sweat glands produce water for evaporation. Note that this is activated only when water evaporation and heat loss from the blood are insufficient to cool the body adequately
Arrector pili muscles contract, erecting hairs and increasing the thermal insulation of the skin	Arrector pili muscles relaxed, lowering hairs and reducing the thermal insulation of the skin

Adapted from Herlihy and Maebius (2000).

Nutrient storage

Deep-seated areas of the dermis contain lipids in adipose tissue, in which vitamin D_2 is synthesized in the presence of sunlight, which is needed for absorption of calcium and phosphorus (Herlihy and Maebius 2000).

Sensory reception

Nerve receptors in the skin are sensitive to pain, touch, temperature and pressure. These serve to protect the skin by causing the body to react to painful or unpleasant stimuli. Movement is stimulated by the detection of differences in pressure, e.g. pain, which are transmitted to the brain, where a reflex indicating discomfort directs blood to flow back into the affected area (Herlihy and Maebius 2000).

Communication

Beauty is identified through the skin; scarring can lead to a lowering of self-esteem. Facial expressions of frowning, smiling, pouting and blushing are outward signs of how the person feels. Pheromones are substances secreted by glands in the skin which stimulate the sense of smell and are thought to act as sexual stimulants (Bevan 1978).

Excretion

Skin is able to excrete small amounts of salt, water and waste such as urea (Herlihy and Maebius 2000).

Factors that influence skin characteristics

The quality and function of the skin are significantly affected by increasing age. Ultraviolet (UV) radiation can have a range of harmful effects on the skin, from making it tough and leathery to damaging the DNA of skin cells resulting in an increased risk of squamous cell carcinoma and malignant melanoma (Herlihy and Maebius 2000). Short-term exposure of lightly pigmented skin to UV radiation can lead to blistering or a second-degree burn (Wysocki 1992). Adequate skin hydration is provided by sebum production and intact skin. Factors that can affect skin hydration include relative humidity, removal of sebum and advancing age (Herlihy and Maebius 2000).

The normal skin pH is acidic, between 4.0 and 5.5 (Berg 1988). Excessive use of alkaline soap, alcohol and acetone can have damaging effects on the quality of skin. Alkaline soap reduces the thickness and number of cell layers in the stratum corneum (White et al. 1987), reduces the water-holding capacity of the skin and increases skin pH, all of which increase the risk of bacterial entry and resistance (Berg 1988). The application of alcohol and acetone to the skin can dehydrate and/or reduce sebum production in the skin (Leyden 1986).

A well-balanced diet of protein, carbohydrate, fat, vitamins and essential minerals is needed to maintain healthy skin. An increase in any of these will not normally improve the condition of skin except when trauma has occurred (Wysocki 2000). Adequate supplies of vitamin C are necessary for collagen formation during healing; fats are needed by cells to form the fatty layer and carbohydrates for extra energy requirements during cell division and for cell metabolism. Vitamins A, B, C, D, iron, zinc and copper are needed to maintain a healthy skin (Wysocki 1992).

Just about every group of drug can affect the condition of the skin from steroid medications that cause thinning of the skin to analgesics and antipsychotic agents. Certain medications cause phototoxicity and photosensitivity (antibiotics, antipsychotic drugs); others interfere with the inflammatory reaction (steroids, non-steroidal anti-inflammatory drugs or NSAIDs) (Wysocki 2000).

The effects of ageing on the skin

All components of the integumentary system are affected as human beings age:

- The sensitivity of the immune system is reduced as a result of the loss of macrophages and other cells of the immune system, which in turn further encourages infection and skin damage. Epidermal cells reproduce more slowly, and are larger and more irregular in shape. These changes result in thinner, more translucent skin (Herlihy and Maebius 2000).
- There is a reduction in sebum secretion and sweating, causing dry, coarse, itchy and scaly skin. There is a marked increase in the incidence of skin problems such as pruritis, dermatitis, squamous cell carcinoma, basal cell carcinoma, blistering diseases, venous leg ulcers and pressure ulcers in elderly people (Tanj and Phillips 2001).
- Less melanin is produced, which results in paler skin and increased sensitivity to the effects of the sun. The increased risk of skin cancer and infection is caused by a decrease in the numbers of Langerhans' cells, which affects the immunocompetence of the skin. Some melanocytes produce extra melanin resulting in 'age spots' in areas exposed to the sun. A reduced inflammatory response may alter allergic reactions and impede the rate of healing. However, in spite of poor healing, the quality of scar tissue is improved in elderly people (Tanj and Phillips 2001).

- As the epidermis thins and sensory receptors diminish in capacity, so the incidence of injuries and infections increases. Older people are more likely to be accidentally burned or injured without realizing (Herlihy and Maebius 2000).
- Sagging and wrinkling appear as skin weakens; the dermis thins by about 20% (Wysocki 1992), collagen is lost and elasticity decreases, particularly in those areas exposed to the sun. Collagen is needed as a foundation for healing in a wound, from which a matrix forms. As the hypodermis becomes thinner people are more prone to pressure damage, bruising and small haemorrhages (Herlihy and Maebius 2000).
- Overheating and increased sensitivity to temperature changes caused by loss of efficiency of the sweat glands and a diminished dermal blood supply may result in a reduction in the ability to lose heat (Herlihy and Maebius 2000).
- Intrinsic ageing is associated with delayed wound healing (Tanj and Phillips 2001). There is slower healing in the older person as epidermal cell turnover time is increased (Wysocki 1992).
- Vascularity decreases in subcutaneous tissue so that drugs administered subcutaneously are absorbed more slowly and healing time is increased. As the vascularity of the sacrum decreases, less external pressure is needed to stop the blood flow than in younger people (Shubert and Heraud 1994).

Types of skin damage

Damage to skin may be precipitated by a number of different factors: mechanical, chemical, vascular, infectious, allergic and thermal, and by radiation and extravasation. Each will result in a different initial response such as the development of erythema, macules, papules, vesicles, erosion or ulcers, and may later develop into more serious secondary lesions (Bryant 1992). Correct recognition of the type of lesion and its cause is essential before treatment is initiated, because different lesions will require different treatment plans.

Chemically induced damage can occur as a result of exposure to incontinence, inappropriate cleansing solutions, improper use of substances such as skin sealants and acidic drainage from fistulae, which erode the surface of the skin (Benbow and Iosson 2002). Vascular damage may manifest as ulcers on the legs or feet caused by venous or arterial insufficiency, neuropathy or a combination of factors. Injury is more probable from minor knocks and healing is usually slow (Herlihy and Maebius 2000).

Infectious lesions may be precipitated by infections with *Candida albicans*, herpes simplex or herpes zoster, or by impetigo; in all cases the underlying cause must be identified and treated. Allergic reactions may develop after exposure to a local skin irritant or allergen such as wound dressing adhesives, local treatments, solutions, or a range of cosmetics, soaps and other everyday substances.

Skin lesions present in many different forms according to the underlying aetiology. The misdiagnosis of skin lesions based on appearance is common. Diagnosis is aided by location, distribution, configuration (the pattern in which the lesions are arranged (Lookingbill and Marks 1993)), morphology (developing or changing nature of a body site (Collins et al. 2002)), the tissue affected and the presence or absence of inflammation. Some of the more common lesions are (Lookingbill and Marks 1993):

- fissure: a thin linear tear in the epidermis
- erosion: wider than a fissure and superficial
- ulcer: a defect causing loss of epidermis and all or part of the dermis
- atrophy: loss of skin tissue leading to wrinkling of the epidermis and/or the dermis
- weals (hives): papules or plaques of dermal oedema with central pallor and irregular borders
- telangiectasia: superficial blood vessels enlarged so that they are clinically visible
- cyst: a nodule filled with liquid or semi-solid, expressible material
- vesicles and bullae: blisters filled with clear fluid – vesicles < 0.5 cm and bullae > 0.5 cm in diameter
- induration: dermal thickening resulting in skin that feels thicker and firmer than normal.

These are a few of the many lesions that may be seen in practice.

Injury and repair

The ability of skin to regenerate and replace lost epidermal and dermal cells can be a slow process when large areas are damaged with the constant risk of fluid loss and infection. Deliberate incisional wounds with little tissue loss heal relatively quickly with minimal loss of function compared with wounds such as deep abrasions or ulceration where there is extensive tissue loss.

Elderly people, in particular, need good skin care when the skin's resistance to normal wear and tear is reduced because the skin is drier, more easily damaged and slower to heal, added to which there is an altered early inflammatory response (Tanj and Phillips 2001). The speed and quality of wound healing are affected by the quantity and distribution of growth factors in ageing skin (Ashcroft et al. 1997a). Oestrogen is believed to be involved in increasing the rate of wound healing, possibly by stimulating the production of certain growth factors (Ashcroft et al. 1997b).

Excess exposure to UV radiation increases the risk of melanoma and accelerates visible ageing of the skin (Lookingbill and Marks 1993). An obvious solution is to avoid exposure to natural sunlight but the social pressures associated with a tan implying good health and attractiveness prevail, in spite of health education to the contrary.

Care of the skin

Skin is constantly exposed to all kinds of external harmful insults: the drying effects of soap and water, the damaging effects of UV radiation and trauma. Preservation of the production of natural oils in the skin should be a priority. Soap is alkaline so it is preferable to use an alternative for skin cleansing, particularly for patients who are incontinent. There is a strong association between incontinence and the development of pressure ulceration in adults (Barbenel et al. 1977), although there is no proof that incontinence causes pressure ulcers. The skin becomes macerated and fragile with constant exposure to urine and faeces; ammonia is produced by the breakdown of urea and is responsible for the familiar dermatitis excoriation (damage to the surface of the skin caused by physical abrasion such as scratching or dragging a patient over the sheet) (Rainey 2002). Often the result is well-meant recommendations by nurses, doctors and pharmacists to apply a vast array of barrier creams and ointments without any evidence for their effectiveness. The problem is compounded by the application of layer after layer of cream without adequate washing in between. Proprietary skin cleansers are available that are pH balanced and combine emollient, water repellent, deodorant and a barrier. Cleansing is easier because the foam loosens and lifts soiling from the skin, no water is needed and the skin is left clean and moisturized. Cooper and Gray (1998) found significant cost savings associated with the use of a skin cleanser in a randomized trial as well as reduced skin breakdown and irritation in a group of incontinent patients.

Emollients used in place of soap can soothe and hydrate the skin for short periods. A lipid film is provided by the emollient on contact with the skin which traps water in the stratum corneum of the epidermis, allowing the cells to swell and restore the skin's permeability barrier and flexibility (Crawford 1999). Other advantages associated with the use of emollients include a steroid-sparing effect (a reduction of 75% in the use of topical steroids was demonstrated by Marhle et al. (1989)) and a direct anti-inflammatory effect by preventing the penetration of irritants and allergens (Cork 1997). Emollients are available as bath and shower additives, ointments or creams; however, their action is short-lived. The application of a lanolin-free cream or ointment after cleansing is recommended to preserve the quality of the skin (Hampton and Collins 2001). Care must be taken when the preparation contains preservatives to extend the shelf-life of the product: they may cause allergic skin reactions or sensitivity. The application and reapplication of creams until they clog, particularly in skin creases, and hairy and moist areas, should also be avoided. The value of applying barrier creams and ointments is currently under review (M Clark, personal communication).

Maceration or excoriation of the skin may occur as a result of prolonged contact with urine and/or faeces or other moisture, causing interference with the protective ability of the skin. In practice, overhydration will increase the risk of damage from bacteria and trauma because it makes the skin more fragile. Effective prevention of excoriation can be achieved by using a special skin barrier cream, which should be applied prophylactically when damage is expected, e.g. in the sacral area, from incontinence. Protection for skin that is already damaged can be achieved using a barrier film. Care must be taken not to rub the skin of vulnerable patients vigorously, as advocated by Hughes (1989), because it is now known that vigorous rubbing can cause superficial and deep tissue damage (Olsen et al. 1992). Underhydration of skin caused by general dehydration will have significant effects on the flexibility of the tissues, increasing the effects of relatively minor injury in the skin of elderly people (Herlihy and Maebius 2000).

Implications for practice

Skin conditions in the UK are many and varied and constitute a major drain on NHS resources. In a 1992 survey (British Association of Dermatologists 1993), 3% of adults claimed to have had a skin complaint within the previous 7 days. In the same survey it was found that about 10% of primary health-care consultations are skin related, although an estimated 75% of people with skin conditions are not seen by a doctor. Skin cancer is the most common cancer; more than 30 000 cases are diagnosed each year with the incidence of malignant melanoma doubling every 10–15 years (British Association of Dermatologists 1993). It can be seen from these figures that skin problems are common and they demand huge resources for consultations and treatment. The best advice for preserving skin integrity is to keep it simple – prevent skin problems. Patient and health-care staff education is vital to ensure speedy and appropriate treatment. Skin should be kept clean and free of clogging creams and ointments unless there is solid rationale for their use.

Student exercises

- Which layer of the epidermis forms the cuticle?
- What is the difference between the apocrine and the eccrine glands?
- Explain the relationship between vasoconstriction and vasodilatation in body temperature regulation.
- What are the four types of heat loss from the skin?
- How does ageing affect the skin?
- Examine your own skin care practices and compare with what is best practice.

CHAPTER THREE

What is a wound?

Introduction to the general principles of wound management

After assessment of the patient and correction or alleviation of those conditions that are known to interfere with healing, an accurate, comprehensive wound assessment by a trained nurse is the next vital prerequisite to successful healing. This assessment will provide baseline information about the current state of the wound, which should then ensure that appropriate measures are implemented to aid healing.

This chapter focuses on the various clinical appearances of wounds and their management; however, it should be remembered that wounds are difficult to categorize. They often present with various mixtures of slough, necrotic tissue, granulating tissue and epithelializing tissue in their base or surface. Clear, accurate, regular documentation will assist in assessing the progress of healing and evaluation of the appropriateness of management.

Types of wounds

A wound is defined as a breach in the epidermis or dermis that initiates a process of repair, which can be related to trauma or pathological changes within the skin or the body (Davis et al. 1992, Collins et al. 2002). Wounds may be either acute – wounds that are healing as anticipated – or chronic in nature (e.g. pressure ulcers) – wounds that are failing to heal as anticipated or that have become fixed in any one phase of wound healing for a period of 6 weeks (Collier 2002).

Collier (2003) believes that all wounds can be classified into one of the following categories:

- mechanical: e.g. surgical/traumatic wounds
- chronic: e.g. leg ulcers/pressure ulcers

- burns, chemical or thermal injuries: may be further classified by depth of injury
- malignant: primary lesions such as melanomas.

The acute wound

An acute wound is a recently inflicted wound that will usually heal without problems, providing the appropriate measures are taken to reduce the risk of infection and support wound healing. In acute wounds, the cell membranes may be disrupted, causing acute tissue damage to the skin and underlying tissues, in several ways. Skin may be cut (laceration), torn, burst or crushed (avulsion injury) by external forces. Other physical insults may include intentional surgery, infection (abscess), extreme heat (burns, scalds), subzero cold (chilblains), vascular interruption, chemical attack, bites or high-voltage electricity, all of which may result in the production of non-viable tissue.

The chronic wound

A chronic wound is one that has remained unhealed for more than 6 weeks with complex and multiple factors that impede healing (Collins et al. 2002).

Chronic wounds are costly and labour intensive to treat over long periods of time. Examples of chronic wounds are leg ulcers (of varying aetiology), pressure ulcers, malignant wounds and diabetic foot ulcers. In all cases of chronic wounds a predisposing factor(s) is responsible for impairing the ability of the body to maintain tissue integrity or heal the wound. Examples of predisposing medical conditions include impaired venous drainage and arterial supply, metabolic abnormalities, unrelieved mechanical forces, malignant disease and genetic disorders. Frequently, in elderly people, several predisposing factors that interfere with wound healing are found in the same individual at the same time. The key issue is to identify and to correct or modify the underlying cause(s) at an early stage to allow healing to occur.

The process of normal wound healing

The aim of healing can be regarded as life preserving, not just a function of regeneration and restoration of tissue integrity so that the wound remains uninfected, heals with a minimum of scar tissue and becomes functional again. It is an extremely complex process that proceeds through a series of well-ordered cellular and biochemical events, with many factors that have favourable or unfavourable influence (Westaby 1985). In healthy adults and children wound healing does not pose too much of a problem; wounds heal quickly, usually without incident even with a minor degree of infection. As people age, however, wound healing becomes more problematic, with even minor wounds proving to be challenging and with the process proving difficult to control.

Wound closure

Healing by primary intention

Deliberate incisional wounds with no tissue loss, where the wound edges are held in apposition to each other, will heal by primary intention (Dealey 2000). However, the phases of the healing process will progress in the same order as in a chronic or slow healing wound. During the first 24 hours a mild inflammatory reaction occurs with fluid and cellular exudate being produced; often the patient will be slightly pyrexial and the wound edges will be swollen, red and warm. After 2–3 days epithelial cells will have bridged the gap between the wound edges and helped to seal it. The collagen network forms over the next 10 days and regeneration begins. Sutures can usually be removed in 5–10 days but healing continues for much longer. A thin white scar may be all that remains after 6 months as the tissues shrink, and become paler and less vascular.

Secondary intention healing

Healing by secondary intention occurs when damage has resulted in loss of tissue and where the skin edges cannot be brought together for wound closure. Chronic wounds such as pressure ulcers, leg ulcers and dehisced surgical wounds heal by secondary intention. This is a protracted process because aggravating factors that have predisposed to the initial wound are still present, e.g. in the patient with a pressure ulcer overlying his right hip – the side he favours lying on – healing will not succeed if he is allowed to continue to lie on the right side; inadequate nutritional status in a patient with a dehisced wound will not support healing. The wound with large amounts of tissue loss will take from months to years to heal because the defect must be filled with scar tissue then covered with epithelial tissue. Healing time is also dependent on the size and location of the wound.

Tertiary intention healing

Wounds managed by delayed closure are classified as healing by tertiary intention or delayed primary closure. Wounds allowed to heal in this way are usually dehisced abdominal wounds complicated by infection (Waldrop and Doughty 2000). Where there is significant bacterial contamination in the wound, the superficial layers are left open and packed lightly with dressings. The body cavity is sealed to prevent evisceration. Over 4–5 days the wound develops resistance to infection and is closed with the minimum amount of suture material and lower risk of infection (Westaby 1985).

The stages of normal wound healing

The stages of wound healing have been described in various different ways but all follow a similar course of events whether the wound is acute or chronic. Variations in the length of time a wound takes to heal are dependent on the degree of tissue damage, cause of the wound, general condition of the patient and ongoing management of care.

Dealey (2000, p. 2) describes the healing process as a series of highly complex, interdependent and overlapping stages. At present clinicians can observe changes only at a macroscopic level and much of what happens at the microscopic level has yet to be discovered (Harding 1996).

Healing occurs as a result of a very efficient and vigorous form of intensive care carried out by teams of cells with distinct roles to play. There are four main phases of healing:

1. the acute inflammatory phase
2. the destructive phase
3. the proliferative phase
4. the maturation phase (Kindlen and Morison 1997).

Which are involved in the healing of all soft tissue injuries? Healing is said to be complete when the skin surface has re-formed and the skin has regained most of its tensile strength (Davis et al. 1992).

The acute inflammatory phase of healing (0–3 days)

Initiation of the clotting cascade is the first requirement or reaction to damage to blood vessels after injury. The aims are to control cellular injury, contain blood loss and prepare a clean wound bed for repair (Waldrop and Doughty 2000). On injury the blood vessels are disrupted and deeper layers of tissue exposed; the injured cells release clotting factors that direct the activities concerned with haemostasis. There is a brief period of vasoconstriction to conserve blood loss, with the clot serving to act as a temporary bacterial barrier and a framework for migrating cells. The breakdown of the platelets in the wound releases a mixture of growth factors that attracts the necessary components for repair to proceed, so clotting functions as an essential first step in the healing process.

Three components interact in clot formation: the damaged vessel wall, platelets and coagulation factors. When damage occurs a series of processes is triggered which result in the release of a number of chemical mediators (mediators are chemical substances that influence the activity of cells, acting as local messengers) and intercell messenger substances called cytokines, which in turn lead to a complex cycle of events resulting in haemostasis and healing. The clotting cascade is a finely tuned series of events that results in a temporary plug of platelets forming at the site of vessel injury to limit immediate blood loss; the platelets also release serotonin and vasoconstrictors. When the clot has served its purpose it is lysed by plasmin (Kindlen and Morison 1997).

Following this part of the process there is vasodilatation, enhanced vessel permeability, increased collagen synthesis by fibroblasts and chemotaxis of macrophages. Macrophages are large, mobile, phagocytic cells, which are not a component of blood but play a vital role in inflammation and initiate angiogenesis (the process by which new blood vessels are formed). Macrophages, with monocytes and lymphocytes, take over the orchestration of the activities within the wound and coordinate the processes that follow. Macrophages are responsible for:

- attracting fibroblasts into the wound and their multiplication
- stimulating fibroblasts to produce collagen and ground substance
- manufacturing proteins, enzymes and other substances
- breaking down various complex molecules into simple sugars and amino acids to provide local nutrition.

Macrophages are considered to be the local biochemical control centres for healing (Wall 1985).

Chemical mediators, some of which may be inhibitory and others stimulatory, regulate healing. The purpose of the inflammatory phase of healing is to prepare the injured tissues for the subsequent phases of healing. Histamine and other mediators are released from the damaged cells and white blood cells are attracted to the site of injury via locally dilated blood vessels, causing the familiar signs of inflammation: redness, heat, swelling, pain, loss of function and oedema (Kindlen and Morison 1997).

Neutrophil leukocytes may be regarded as the first line of defence against infection at the wound site because they are actively phagocytic. Unfortunately, in elderly people, as a result of diabetes mellitus, debility or steroid medication or in people with a failing immune system, this response can be depressed, making the early detection of infection more difficult. The overall function of inflammation is to neutralize and destroy any toxic agents at the site of an injury and to restore tissue homoeostasis (Collier 2003).

The inflammatory stage of healing usually lasts between 4 and 5 days, after which time the blood vessels return to normal dimensions, the signs of inflammation subside and the fibroblasts infiltrate to help to reconstruct the tissue.

The function of this phase of healing is to clear the site of injury of dead and devitalized tissue through the action of macrophages, which are able to destroy bacteria and produce growth factors that stimulate the formation of fibroblasts, the synthesis of collagen and the process of angiogenesis (Kindlen and Morison 1997). Cellular activity is optimal at normal body temperature with any deviation from the norm adversely affecting the process (Dealey 2000).

The inflammatory stage of healing is complex and demanding on body resources and energy, so any patient-related factors that prolong the inflammatory stage of healing would weaken the patient and delay healing.

The destructive phase of healing (2–6 days)

At this stage the nature of the active cell population changes to clear devitalized tissue from the wounded area. Neutrophils and macrophages are the cells responsible for clearing the wound site of devitalized and unwanted material. Macrophages assume control of the operation and serve several important functions. Adequate numbers of macrophages are vital at this stage to engulf and digest bacteria, remove excess fibrin and produce growth factors, because they attract more macrophages to, and stimulate the production of, fibroblasts in the wound site. If the supply of macrophages reduces, healing will cease (Kindlen and Morison 1997).

Fibroblasts are the cells responsible for most collagen, elastin and fibronectin synthesis; they give strength and structure to the repair and have a large role to play in wound healing. Their numbers increase when wounds are present and they respond to chemotactic stimuli. Fibroblasts stimulate cell migration, angiogenesis, embryonic development and wound healing, and are involved in soft tissue growth and regeneration (Collins et al. 2002). Collagen, the most abundant protein in the animal world, is responsible for holding the body together and is laid down and modified during the proliferative and maturation stages of healing (Collins et al. 2002).

A specialized mobile form of fibroblast known as a myofibroblast is responsible for pulling the healing tissues in the wound contraction stage of healing to reduce the size of the wound (Collins et al. 2002). The focus has now switched to repair and the production of new collagen-rich (scar) tissue through intense cellular activity.

The proliferative phase of healing (3–24 days)

At this stage newly forming capillaries infiltrate the wound site to nourish and support the development of connective tissue, a process called angiogenesis. It can take 7–10 days for the formation of granulation tissue and the next stage of healing: the proliferative phase. However, during this time, the base of the wound may be irregular and covered with slough or necrotic material (Harding 1996). Granulation tissue consists of a network of new blood vessels in a collagen-rich matrix that fills the base of a wound. Granulation tissue is very fragile and can be recognized as the bright-red granular tissue in a wound. A range of growth factors stimulates nourishment. Growth factors are a subclass of cytokines (biological factors), comprising proteins, thought to direct several biological processes including wound repair, such as growth and differentiation of cells. More than 20 growth factors have been identified, their function being to stimulate specific physiological activities in particular cells (Collins et al. 2002). Cytokines also contribute to the regulation of cellular function and wound repair (Waldrop and Doughty 2000).

The extracellular matrix (ECM) or ground substance of connective tissue consists of water, glycosaminoglycans (e.g. hyaluronic acid) and proteins, and can influence the behaviour of cells (Collins et al. 2002); it is said to regulate cell-to-cell communication (Kindlen and Morison 1997). Communication is necessary to shape and direct the orientation of the parts that make up the healing tissue. Over a number of weeks, the proliferative phase consists of active granulation and contraction working in concert to fill the dead space of the wound, strengthen it and make it shrink by contraction (Harding 1996).

The maturation phase of healing (3 weeks to months or years)

This is the phase in which the wound becomes covered with new skin (re-epithelialization) and there is tissue contraction and re-organization of the healing tissue within the wound. Epithelial cells that have remained around the remnants of hair follicles, sebaceous and sweat glands, and the wound margins divide and migrate over the granulation tissue. The conditions at the wound site must be conducive to easy movement of the epithelial cells, i.e. warm and moist (Winter 1962), otherwise the production of eschar will impede the speed of movement and slow healing down. The myofibroblasts contract to decrease the size of the wound and bring the edges together. The wound changes colour from red to white as the temporarily increased vascularity of the wound subsides. Wound strength increases as the collagen fibres are re-organized but the resulting scar tissue is never as strong as the original tissue (Kindlen and Morison 1997).

Presenting wound healing in four phases suggests that it is very straight-forward and proceeds without problems. When assessing a wound it is frequently difficult to identify which stage of healing it has reached as a result of a mixture of appearances within the same wound, e.g. the granu-lating wound may have areas of slough present suggesting that the inflammatory phase has not completed its job of cleaning the wound of devitalized tissue. Most frequently, the stages of the healing process overlap and may not reflect the age of the wound as a result of intrinsic or extrinsic factors affecting the rate of healing.

This section has described the normal phases of the healing process that will apply, whether it is an incised wound or an open wound healing by sec-ondary intention. The time it takes will vary according to the amount of tissue loss, age of the patient and other factors affecting the rate of healing. In an incised wound less energy and activity are seen than in an open wound and the healing time is minimal as a result of the small amount of tissue loss. The inflammatory phase allows the macrophages rapidly to summon macrophages, growth factors and fibroblasts to the injured area. The endothelial cells of healthy capillaries start to grow and 'bud' and grow into the wound space to form new capillaries, and eventually draw and seal the wound edges together.

In an open wound, the same processes happen but they heal by the formation of granulation tissue in all dimensions of the wound. Healing begins in the same way, but a thin zone of inflammation persists in the sur-face layer of granulation tissue, which advances as the capillaries regenerate and grow. Fibroblasts synthesize large quantities of collagen and ground substance which form the advancing front of healing tissue. Eventually granulation tissue fills the defect and epithelialization occurs (Wall 1985).

Implications for practice

During the vital inflammatory phase of healing, certain impediments may affect the process, either to delay or to prevent it, such as the presence of a foreign body or devitalized tissue, the inappropriate use of cleansing solutions or continued mechanical trauma (Kindlan and Morison 1997). Patients with compromised immune responses, those on steroids, or those who are malnourished or dehydrated will experience delayed healing or non-healing of wounds.

Wound surfaces must be kept warm, moist and clean, so if they are left exposed for long periods they will become cold, dry and possibly contam-inated. The cooling effects from exposure or cold cleansing solutions on cell metabolism are particularly detrimental to healing progress; poor tissue perfusion, hypoxia and chemical agents may also be responsible for impeding healing.

Newly formed granulation tissue is extremely fragile and easily damaged by the removal of adherent dressings; these should be avoided. This phase of healing is dependent on adequate supplies of nutrients such as vitamin C, iron, protein and oxygen, and can be delayed with increasing age (Kindlan and Morison 1997). Care to avoid local trauma from dressings and incorrect management is the key to supporting, promoting and protecting the still fragile, newly epithelialized wound.

The systemic effects of wound healing

There is a necessary interdependence between the systemic response, which maintains homoeostasis, to the presence of a wound and the wound itself. Wounds will not heal unless the necessary components are supplied and delivered to the cells that require them. It is a well-recognized phenomenon that tissues with poor blood supply heal more slowly and are more easily infected. The patient may be taking an adequate and nutritious diet but, if the nutrients cannot be delivered to the site of injury, because of impaired vascularity, healing will not occur. Wound healing is a major challenge, e.g. to patients with diseased blood vessels such as people with diabetes and atherosclerosis or the young smoker with Buerger's disease whose diet is adequate but who has non-healing, gangrenous ulceration in his lower extremity. The site of damage, blood supply, presence of haematoma, and general physical and psychological condition of the patient are some of the factors that influence the rate of healing.

Damaged tissue is very fragile and therefore needs careful handling. Minor injury can be compounded by the way the wound is managed, causing further damage to blood vessels and disrupting vascular supply, leading to tissue hypoxia, increased healing demands and subsequent delayed healing.

Surgical stress induces profound peripheral vasoconstriction of the subcutaneous and skin blood vessels supplying peripheral tissues (Rowell 1986) by activating the autonomic nervous system. In turn these effects will reduce the amount of available nutrients and oxygen to the wound site.

Cold, pain, fear, smoking and certain pharmacological preparations will act as sympathetic nervous system activators, adversely influencing healing. These should be addressed, i.e. keep the patient warm and prevent heat loss, control pain, reduce anxiety and fear, discontinue β-blockers and encourage smoking cessation (West and Gimbel 2000).

Westaby (1985) describes a phenomenon whereby early hypovolaemic shock caused by trauma or surgery will rapidly lead to reduced perfusion at the edges of a surgical wound, even before the clinical signs of shock are evident. At the point of shock, blood is not fully restored to the wound edges, which may lead to wound dehiscence and delayed healing.

Starved, poorly perfused surgical patients heal more slowly and, the better the general condition of the patient, the better the state of the wound. Malnutrition may be precipitated by, e.g. extended periods of starvation resulting from surgery, after trauma, malignancy, malabsorptive bowel conditions or fistulae, all of which will reduce the patient's ability to heal and cause increased susceptibility to infection.

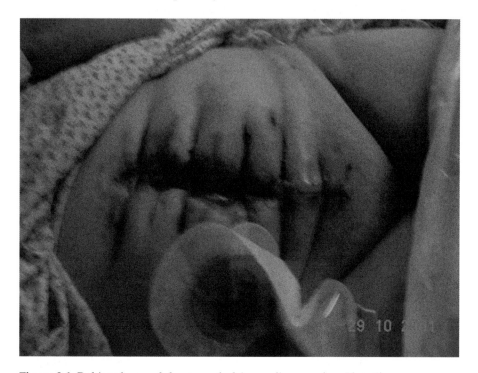

Figure 3.1 Dehisced wound due to underlying malignancy (see Plate 1).

The healed wound

The wound is, therefore, healed when epithelialization resurfaces the damaged area. Epithelial cells, under the right conditions, multiply and migrate across the surface from the wound margins in a partial-thickness wound and from remnants of hair follicles in a superficial wound. The size of the wound reduces, controlled by a complex set of mechanisms that halt the process at the appropriate stage. The result is newly formed, fragile tissue that is easily disrupted (Davis et al. 1992). Factors that will impede epithelialization include variations in temperature and pH, the presence of foreign material, desiccation and infection. A major culprit is the nurse carrying out unnecessarily frequent dressing changes or applying adherent dressings.

During the maturation stage of healing, shortening or contraction of scar tissue may occur due to re-organization of collagen which can restrict movement and cause tightness, with growth and development being affected in children. Surgery may be necessary to release and graft affected areas.

In full-thickness wounds the process of healing continues for some time after epithelialization with further re-organization, differentiation and re-modelling to strengthen the healed tissue. However, healed or scar tissue will never be as strong as the original tissue.

Keloid scarring forms when the control of proliferation and maturation is disrupted, producing a hard, raised and possibly painful or pruritic area, which often extends into undamaged areas. Excision of keloid scarring does not usually result in improvement.

Moist wound healing

The traditional method for encouraging wounds to heal was to allow them to dry out and form a scab, believing that the scab would protect the damaged area. The theory of moist wound healing evolved in the 1960s when Winter (1962) found that superficial wounds in pigs, covered with polythene, healed nearly twice as quickly as those left to dry and scab. The polythene retained moisture in contact with the wound supporting epithelial cell migration. Concerns about the increased risk of infection in a moist wound were allayed when Hutchinson and Lawrence (1991) demonstrated that occluded wounds showed a lower infection rate. The theory of moist wound healing led to the development of many of the modern-day occlusive dressings that provide a moist healing environment.

The benefits of moist wound healing are as follows (Field and Kerstein 1994):

- less reported pain: free nerve endings are bathed in physiological fluids
- fewer infections reported: viable host defences, less dry, dead tissue to harbour micro-organisms
- less injury on removal: moist wound-healing interface
- less risk of micro-organism transfer: less airborne dispersal of micro-organisms on removal
- efficient autolytic débridement versus mechanical for traditional drying dressings: enzymes require water for hydrolysis of proteins.

The environment under the dressing

Dressings provide a physical barrier to protect the wound from the external environment, retain moisture and exudate factors, and insulate the wound to reduce heat loss (Davis et al. 1992). Modern synthetic dressings provide a wider range of useful properties than those made from traditional gauze and cotton-wool materials. Vapour permeability is a key factor in modern dressings to allow transmission of water vapour (and gases) through the dressing and away from the wound to reduce maceration. The surface must be kept moist but not wet. Film dressings, for example, are permeable to water vapour and gases but not to water or bacteria; hydrocolloid dressings are impermeable to water, gases and bacteria, and insulate the wound; an hypoxic environment is created which promotes angiogenesis.

If a wound is left to dry out, desiccation will happen and a scab or crust will form made up of cellular debris and protein. By applying an occlusive or semi-occlusive dressing the wound surface will remain moist, precluding scab formation and facilitating the migration of cells in the epidermis and dermis. If a scab is allowed to form, it will impede the movement of epithelial cells, causing them to penetrate to a lower, moister level in the wound to multiply, which will take more time and energy and, ultimately, delay healing.

Gauze was traditionally used to absorb fluid, wick it away from the wound and then allow it to evaporate. However, there are problems associated with the presence of exudate in the dressing relating to the attraction and passage of bacteria through the dressing to the wound surface. This is known as 'strike-through' and indicates that the dressing is ready to be changed. The collection of fluid under a dressing will very quickly cause maceration if the dressing is not changed. Modern wound dressings, with their properties of vapour permeability, balance the rate of vapour passage (transpiration) to reduce the risk of maceration and leakage, and extend the life of the dressing. Extending the dressing wear time is, in turn, important to reduce interference with the healing wound. Accurate assessment of exudate levels influences both the choice of dressing and the frequency of change.

A wound that contains necrotic or sloughy tissue must be débrided or de-sloughed before granulation tissue can form. The application of hydro-gel, hydrocolloid and film dressings will de-slough or débride the wound effectively. They work through the natural process of autolysis within the moist environment to re-hydrate necrotic tissue to facilitate its removal.

Benefits to patients

Practical benefits of modern dressings afforded to patients include:

- ease of application: a single nurse can cope with applying most modern dressings
- longer duration of time in place: some up to 7–14 days

- flexibility to conform to difficult areas of the body and easier movement when in place
- protection from external contamination such as bacteria, faeces and urine
- allow the patient to shower or bath without getting the wound wet or needing a dressing change.

Conclusion

Wounds will heal only if the local and systemic conditions are conducive to healing. A well-nourished, young, healthy person with a wound will normally heal without problems whereas wound healing in an elderly, malnourished, ill person will present major challenges to the practitioner.

Student exercises

- Examine the reasons why a deep wound will take longer to heal than a superficial wound.
- Consider the systemic effects of illness on wound healing.

CHAPTER FOUR

The patient with a wound

The wound care practice of nurses has been described as 'outdated, ritualistic and lacking in foundation in fact or research' and that it could ultimately provide evidence for cases of malpractice in court (Walsh and Ford 1989). Castledine (1992) stated: 'it is dangerous for a nurse to perform a dressing change without proper education, preparation and experience and it is also upsetting for the patient'. Recognition of the need for more research evidence to underpin practice is a move in the right direction but even today there are many questionable practices being undertaken which do not have sound scientific bases. As nurses we have a professional responsibility to update our knowledge in light of new evidence and developments in wound management and to question all we do.

What is needed?

Accurate, comprehensive wound assessment is a vital prerequisite to successful resolution and uncomplicated healing, with the nursing skills required being many and varied. The assessment provides valuable information on which informed decisions about patient and wound management can be made. Documentation of findings from the assessment should be made as succinctly and accurately as possible, to allow consistent management across health-care boundaries such as from primary to secondary care and between different care-givers.

Assessing a patient with a wound

Wound assessment is only one part of the total patient assessment which will include assessment of, for example, level of mobility, degree of dependence, nutritional status, the presence or absence of concurrent illness such as diabetes, anaemia, carcinoma, cardiovascular or peripheral vascular disease, mental state and attitude to having a wound, to mention a few. Recognition of those factors that will delay or indeed promote the healing process should also direct patient and wound management. Problems associated with a person's physical or psychological states which are known to impede healing should be identified and dealt with as far as possible. Contrary to the belief of many nurses, successful wound healing is totally dependent on the innate ability of the individual to heal, not on which dressing is used.

Regular patient and wound assessment will provide baseline data from which treatment decisions are made; however, many wounds heal in spite of professional input rather than as a result of conscientious assessment and high-quality management.

Factors affecting wound healing

There must be adequate supplies of nutrients and oxygen available in the body for cell metabolism and effective waste product removal for a wound to heal at the optimal rate. Healing is a systemic process and will be affected by systemic influences (Waldrop and Doughty 2000). It must, however, be remembered that it is not possible to heal all wounds, so the aim will be palliation of symptoms and improved quality of life for the patient with a wound that is unlikely to heal.

The systemic disease processes that adversely affect metabolism and are likely to delay or prevent wound healing are many and varied and include:

* anaemia
* arteriosclerosis
* cancer
* cardiovascular disorders
* diabetes
* immune disorders
* inflammatory diseases
* jaundice, liver failure
* rheumatoid arthritis
* uraemia.

The factors that adversely affect healing can be divided into general factors (e.g. the age of the patient) and local factors (e.g. mechanical stress).

General factors

* age of the patient
* age of the wound

- oxygen deficit and anaemia
- reduced or compromised vascularity
- smoking
- congenital defects
- metabolic disease, e.g. diabetes mellitus
- jaundice
- malignant disease
- nutritional deficiencies
- fluid intake
- medication
- stress, anxiety and sleep disturbances.

Age of the patient

Children heal more quickly and produce stronger scar tissue than elderly people, who may have a multiplicity of medical conditions, poor nutritional intake, or systemic or malignant disease, and take medications that interfere with healing. The ageing process produces irreversible changes in skin, underlying tissue and blood vessels that make a person both more vulnerable to injury and less able to cope with healing, e.g. wound dehiscence is up to three times more likely in people over 60 years of age (Davis et al. 1992). Bond (1998) identified that factors such as long-standing chronic disease, drugs, anxiety, depression and radiotherapy will impair appetite and affect healing.

The effects of ageing on skin and wound healing are the following (Herlihy and Maebius 2000):

- Slower epidermal regeneration: this results in a generalized thinning and translucency of skin. The dermis becomes thinner with fewer collagen and elastic fibres resulting in increased fragility of the skin, wrinkles and slower healing.
- Reduced barrier function: decline in the number of Langerhans' cells reduces the protective immune function of skin. Sebaceous gland activity decreases resulting in dry, coarse, itchy skin.
- Diminished blood supply: vascularity of the dermis reduces as a result of fewer blood vessels and arteriosclerotic changes, causing the skin to become more prone to small haemorrhages and pressure ulcers. Drugs administered subcutaneously are absorbed more slowly.
- Reduced strength and elasticity: caused by slower cellular regeneration.
- Increased sensitivity: caused by the reduction in nerve endings.

Wounds in elderly people will heal with a good cosmetic result in most cases, but it may take longer (Davis et al. 1992).

Age of the wound

Long-standing or chronic wounds are likely to heal slowly. Proteases are enzymes produced by cells that are responsible for breaking down proteins, with their action being closely regulated during wound healing. In chronic wound healing, the level of proteases is higher and persists for longer than in acute wounds. This has a detrimental effect on growth factors that are degraded by proteases, which, in turn, leads to delayed healing. As a result of abnormal activity of inflammatory cytokines, the inflammatory response is prolonged and contributes to delayed healing (Cullen 2001). Much of the current wound healing-related research is focusing on the constituents of acute wound fluid compared with those of chronic wound fluid. This is to try to identify the components that are either deficient or excessive in chronic wound fluid, to try to correct any imbalances. It is thought that, if the properties of acute wound fluid can be reproduced and introduced into chronic wound fluid, these wounds will heal (Wall 2001).

Oxygen deficit and anaemia

'Oxygenation fuels the cellular function essential to the repair process' (Waldrop and Doughty 2000). Reduced oxygen tension is the measure for predicting the potential for wound healing in patients with arterial insufficiency; the normal value for oxygen tension is 5.3 kPa (40 mmHg). Frequently, anaemia is a sign of other disease processes that can adversely affect wound healing alone, e.g. malignancy, malnutrition. Whatever is causing the anaemia, the result will be a reduction in the blood's oxygen-carrying capacity, which means that the oxygen requirements of the cell for metabolism will not be met. Oxygen also plays a vital role at specific stages of the healing process: in the formation of collagen and new capillaries, in epithelial repair and in the control of infection (La Van and Hunt 1990). Chronic anaemia and acute blood loss as in hypovolaemia will seriously affect the ability of the wound to heal (Kindlen and Morison 1997). Other medical conditions, such as chronic obstructive pulmonary disease, will reduce the amount of available oxygen to the tissues.

Reduced or compromised vascularity

Tissue oxygen levels are dependent on adequate perfusion through the tissues as well as adequate oxygenation of the blood. Possible causes of impaired blood flow to the wound area include pressure, arterial occlusion or prolonged vasoconstriction resulting from vascular disease or arteriosclerosis.

Smoking

Smokers and non-smokers regularly exposed to cigarette smoke (Siana et al. 1992) are adversely affected by the nicotine and carbon monoxide they inhale. Carbon monoxide binds to haemoglobin in place of oxygen, significantly reducing the amount of circulating oxygen, which can impede healing. The nicotine absorbed from cigarette smoking causes the peripheral blood flow to be depressed by at least 50% for more than an hour after smoking just one cigarette (Siana et al. 1992). Problems associated with inhibition of epithelialization and scarring have been identified. However, more research is needed to elicit the direct effect of nicotine on wound healing.

Congenital defects

The whole process of wound healing can break down if just one element of the complex sequence of events involved in wound healing is missing. There are a number of congenital diseases that can cause malfunction or failure of healing at various stages. The following are examples of such rare diseases:

* haemophilia: missing clotting factor
* Christmas disease: missing clotting factor
* chronic granulomatous disease: faulty bone marrow gene, which means that neutrophils, responsible for killing bacteria and fungi, do not function correctly
* thrombocytopenia: a decrease in the number of platelets in the blood resulting in the potential for increased bleeding and decreased ability to clot.

Metabolic disease

In patients with well-controlled diabetes mellitus, healing does not present too many problems. There is a high incidence of necrosis and ulceration of the extremities found in people with diabetes who are ageing and have poorly controlled diabetes, often resulting in poor or non-healing wounds, infection and amputation. This is the result of a combination of factors: atherosclerosis (reducing tissue perfusion), neuropathy (loss of sensation), failure to heed the warning signs of impaired healing, and neglect of injuries and infections. Susceptibility to infection is much higher in people with diabetes than in those who are not diabetic (Wall 1985). The initial inflammatory response is weaker where glycosuria is present, with fewer macrophages causing delayed healing and suggesting a form of impaired immunity. Collagen synthesis and deposition are reduced; the final wound strength is reduced and leukocyte function is impaired in relation to the imbalance of glycaemic control.

Jaundice

The risk of wound dehiscence is increased 12-fold when jaundice is present, especially in association with malignant disease (Irvin et al. 1978). Vitamin K and antibiotic prophylaxis are recommended for patients who have jaundice (Wall 1985).

Malignant disease

The link between malignant disease and delayed healing appears to be related to reduced nutritional status caused by a poor appetite. Altered taste perception leading to reduced appetite and changed eating habits were found in one in four cancer patients (Stubbs 1989).

Nutritional deficiencies

Malnutrition is common in hospitals (McWhirter and Pennington 1994) and can affect wound healing in several ways:

- poor wound healing, reduced tensile strength and increased wound dehiscence (Dickerson 1995)
- increased rate of infection (Dickerson 1995)
- poor quality scarring (Pinchkofsky-Devin 1994)
- susceptibility to pressure ulcer development (Dickerson 1995).

Exton-Smith (1971) explored the issue of malnutrition and divided the causes into primary and secondary:

- primary causes: ignorance, social isolation, physical disability, mental disturbance, iatrogenic disorder and poverty
- secondary causes: impaired appetite, masticatory inefficiency, malabsorption, alcoholism, drugs and increased requirements.

Healing necessitates adequate supplies of protein and calories, plus vitamin C and zinc, in particular. Extra supplies of nutrients are required to compensate for increased energy body demands and protein lost in exudate when a patient has a wound. Protein is needed for the repair and replacement of tissue, carbohydrate for energy which spares protein for healing, vitamin C for collagen synthesis and immunity, vitamin B_{12} for protein synthesis, zinc for protein synthesis and tissue repair, iron for haemoglobin production and copper to increase the tensile strength of the collagen.

Obesity poses major problems relating to wound healing caused by poor vascularity of the tissues and haematoma formation. The presence of obesity does not always equate to good quality, appropriate nutritional intake. Poor nutritional intake may be addressed through supplementation by tablets (e.g. zinc), injection (e.g. vitamins or food supplements) or meal replacements. For those able to take a normal diet, frequent, palatable, high-energy, high-protein foods should be encouraged. Supplementation of vitamin C and zinc is pointless unless there is an identified deficit because these substances cannot be stored in the body.

Uraemia/fluid intake

Adequate intake of fluid (2000–2500 ml/24 h) is essential for efficient cell metabolism and wound healing to compensate for increased demands and excess fluid loss in exudate.

Medication

Sedatives and tranquillizers have the potential to reduce patients' movements, circulation and metabolic function, and reduce their ability to sense and react to stimuli such as excessive pressure or heat. Blood circulation and oxygenation to the periphery are reduced, leading to reduced healing and increased tissue breakdown. Steroids and anti-inflammatory medications interfere with the normal immune response, reducing the inflammatory response, masking signs of infection, suppressing fibroblast and collagen synthesis, and slowing healing down. Cytotoxic medications prolong healing by interfering with cell proliferation and causing immunosuppression, leading to increased infection risk.

Stress, anxiety and sleep disturbance

Psychological problems such as stress and anxiety adversely affect the normal functioning of the immune system (Maier and Laudenslager 1985), leading to sleep disturbance. The body needs time to repair and regenerate (anabolism) during sleep and it has been suggested that healing is promoted by rest and sleep (Adam and Oswald 1983). The patient's altered perception of body image during treatment is associated with stress resulting from the type of treatment, dressings and odours, and after healing, when scarring, the results of surgery, such as amputation or stoma formation, may cause extreme distress.

Local factors

The following are local (or extrinsic) factors that adversely affect wound healing:

- type of wound
- shape of wound
- extent of wound
- temperature
- dressings and inappropriate wound care
- mechanical stress
- foreign bodies
- haematoma
- infection
- radiotherapy
- poor surgical technique
- method of closure of a surgical wound
- inappropriate wound management
- type of tissue in the wound.

Type of wound

Certain wounds will not be expected to heal, e.g. malignant fungating wounds, in which case palliation may be the only option and this should be acknowledged. Most wounds, however, will heal at the optimal rate given the right conditions for healing. Uncomplicated surgical wounds would be expected to heal rapidly, whereas chronic pressure ulcers and wounds with complex underlying pathology will take much longer to heal.

Shape of wound

Uncomplicated, surgically created wounds are likely to heal more rapidly than, e.g., an irregularly shaped, deep pressure ulcer which heals by secondary intention. Drainage of exudate is easier from a surgical wound because it is probably boat shaped with straight sides to facilitate the drainage of exudate, whereas the pressure ulcer may be irregular in shape with undermining and pockets that encourage stasis and retention of exudate. This will increase the infection risk and prove more difficult to dress and manage.

Extent of wound

The size or extent of a wound will influence where the patient is treated, e.g. the patient with extensive burn injuries will need specialized care in a burns unit where expert health-care professionals have the knowledge, experience and expertise to provide the most appropriate high standard of care. Complications of surgical wounds are best treated in hospital where the range of facilities, staff and care is available. Most wounds are moderate to minor and suitable for treatment in the community. Residential care homes and patients at home are served by community nursing services, whereas nursing homes employ qualified nurses. There can often be a gap, however, between the knowledge and skill of nurses if their experience of treating patients with wounds is limited. Fortunately, the number of community tissue viability nurses employed by primary care trusts has grown enormously over recent years to support the care of patients more effectively.

Generally, the larger the wound the longer it will take to heal as a result of increased demands on the body's resources. The wound must be assessed for tunnelling and undermining to ascertain its overall extent and inform predictions of healing time.

Temperature

Vasoconstriction, causing a reduction in the available blood, oxygen and nutrients for cell metabolism, is caused by cold conditions slowing the healing process down. Blood clotting, which is essential for the initiation of healing, fails at very high and very low temperatures, with extremes of heat and cold causing tissue damage. Healing will proceed at the optimal rate in conditions of normothermia (37°C).

Dressings and inappropriate wound care

Broadly, dressing choice should be based on assessment of exudate levels, type of material in the base and sides of the wound, the goals of management and the patient's lifestyle. Dressing choice should also be based on knowledge and experience of the products, the range of presentations, their properties, their mode of action, their limitations and their contraindications.

Mechanical stress

Healing rates are subject to a gradual process which is unique to the individual, but in all cases several months are needed before tissues regain their original strength. Rest and avoidance of excess movement are necessary in the early stages of healing to allow repair and regeneration to begin. Paradoxically, vibrations (continual small movements) have been shown to be helpful in stimulating more rapid reconstruction of bone tissue in healing fractures; the reason for this is not known.

Foreign bodies

Wound contamination, including foreign bodies, soil and bone fragments, suture material and old dressing material, is likely to complicate healing, cause infection and wound breakdown, and ultimately delay healing. The presence of a foreign body or contamination will cause a chronic inflammatory reaction (Westaby 1985), extending that phase of healing and delaying the overall time to healing.

Haematoma

Haematoma is a bruise or collection of blood in the tissues after surgery or trauma and can cause damage in four ways:

1. by exerting pressure on surrounding tissues and capillaries reducing blood flow to the area
2. by a direct toxic effect on tissues
3. by providing a focus for infection through harbouring bacteria
4. by predisposing a wound to dehiscence.

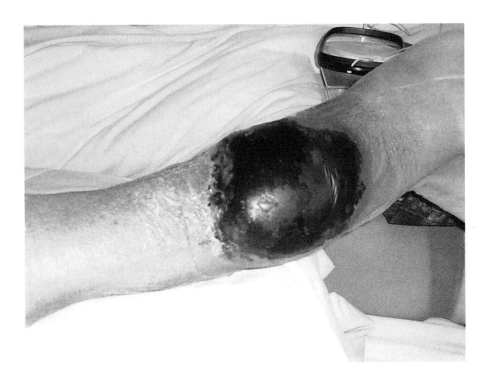

Figure 4.1 Haematoma (see Plate 2).

Infection

Contamination of any wound is almost inevitable as a result of the myriad of organisms present on the skin and in the environment. The body's immune system is capable of dealing with contamination; it is only when the immune system is compromised or overwhelmed that infection strikes. The immune system may be weak or absent as a result of congenital or systemic disease such as cancer, HIV infection, diabetes or anaemia, or immunosuppressant therapy. The problem may arise because the patient is old and/or inadequately nourished.

However, the presence of infection does not necessarily prevent healing, although it can slow it down considerably and cause excessive production of scar tissue. Infection adversely affects healing in the following ways (Davis et al. 1992):

- Infecting organisms compete with the cells in the healing tissue for nutrients and oxygen.
- Infection discourages fibroblast activity and the production of collagen and promotes the release of lysozymes that destroy existing collagen, thus weakening the wound.
- Infection makes additional demands on the inflammatory mechanism and impairs its ability to attend to the wound.
- Abscesses may form in the wound.

Radiotherapy

The response of some fungating wounds to radiotherapy is shrinkage and reduction in exudate production, with a degree of healing at the tumour margins when the bulk of the tumour has decreased (Bale and Jones 1997).

Unfortunately, the effect of the radiotherapy is to prevent or slow down the rate of healing. Radiotherapy can leave the skin and other tissue weakened (Irvin 1981b).

Poor surgical technique

Careful handling of the tissues during surgery will reduce the amount of resultant damage. Rough handling and excessive use of diathermy may cause haematoma formation and devitalize tissues, leading to increased infection risk. Leaving dead space in the surgically created wound should also be avoided.

Method of wound closure

Incorrectly applied wound closure materials can contribute to wound breakdown in already traumatized tissue. They are foreign bodies that can provoke an immune reaction, particularly if they are applied too tightly and cut through the edge of the wound. Bacteria can readily track down the channels made by the closure material.

The following are guidelines for surgeons for closing surgical wounds:

- Choose the right suture for the site of incision, the tensile strength required and the resultant scarring.
- Use an adequate 'bite' when bringing the skin edges together. Larger 'bites' of tissue within the suture will generally result in a stronger wound.
- Choose the appropriate method of suturing. The choice includes:
  - interrupted
  - interrupted – mattress
  - interrupted – subcuticular
  - continuous – blanket
  - continuous – over-and-over.
- Maintain the correct distance evenly between individual sutures.
- Ensure adequate and even tension while suturing – too slack and the wound will not be held together in close approximation, too tight and tissue death may occur (Bale and Jones 1997).

Alternatives to suture materials include clips, staples, skin-closure tapes, butterfly skin closures and semi-occlusive film dressings.

Inappropriate wound management

The use of antiseptic solutions, incorrect dressings, poor dressing technique and lack of knowledge will all adversely affect wound healing.

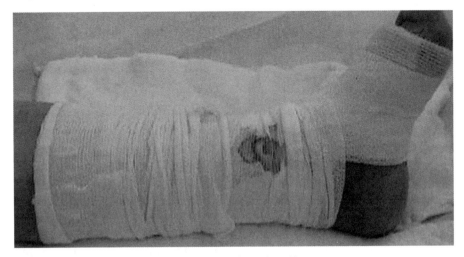

Figure 4.2 An example of poor bandaging (see Plate 3).

Type of tissue in the wound

Some body tissues heal better than others. Bone, parenchymal tissue (liver) and epithelium regenerate well but some more specialized tissues do not heal at all. Cartilage heals very slowly because it consists of collagen, with very few cells and a poor blood supply. The type and colour of material in the wound have significance for management. The aim of wound management is healing but to move a wound from the necrotic stage to the granulating stage is satisfying for the nurse and patient. Recognition of the tissue in the wound will help in devising the treatment plan, e.g. if the wound contains hard, black, necrotic tissue, the aim will be to débride this tissue down to moist, healthy tissue to facilitate the formation of granulation tissue. If surgical débridement is not appropriate, the choice of dressing will focus on rehydrating the devitalized tissue to encourage its separation from viable tissue.

Social factors that may affect healing

Most patients with wounds are treated in the community in either their own homes or residential or nursing homes. Coping with a wound will often require extensive changes to a person's lifestyle for a period of time. Environmental and behavioural factors combined with the availability of, and access to, resources are key considerations in relation to healing a wound. In hospital there is a degree of control over patient management whereas at home the patient will often refuse to comply with advice offered by health-care professionals.

Consideration must be given to the practicality of treatments at home or in nursing or residential care, the ability and motivation of patients to manage themselves, what facilities are available and whether they are prepared to modify their behaviour for the duration of treatment. Clear explanations about the implications of having a wound, what the treatment entails and what is expected of them, as well as how they can be helped, is vital. Explanations about why the patient with a hand injury should rest and elevate the hand to prevent oedema, reduced function and delayed healing should be given so that they take some responsibility for their own care. Advice must be tailored to the injury, the patient and the circumstances.

A realistic plan of care should be developed that fully acknowledges and addresses any fears, objections and reasons for non-compliance, and considers the environment and behaviour. Some patients will need a temporary change of environment until they can cope or increased social services at home; modifications to the home may be necessary. The family, friends and neighbours are often an invaluable source of help. The psychological effects of the injury such as post-traumatic stress disorder, depression, agoraphobia, loss of confidence and personality changes must not be underestimated or neglected.

Political and financial factors that may affect healing

Factors such as time lost from work, inability to return to previous employment or permanent disability can influence both healing and patient compliance. Many people are employed on limited, agency or temporary contracts that do not include payment when absent as a result of sickness, so they fear for their jobs and livelihood. Advice about possible benefits and claims associated with the injury should be obtained from the local benefits agency.

At another level, there are financial implications for the providers of care when decisions have to be made about providing equipment and newer, more expensive dressings. Patients could be potentially disadvantaged where GPs and primary care trusts are unwilling/unable to provide certain treatments and equipment.

Student exercises

- Construct an image of a patient with a number of risk factors for poor wound healing and think about how the problems may be alleviated.
- Consider how the use of information can influence patient compliance with treatment.

CHAPTER FIVE

Diagnosing and assessing wounds

Wounds may be described and documented in many ways but it is not sufficient to record 'wound healing well' or 'wound granulating'; certain relevant aspects of the wound, such as how it looks, if it has changed, its dimensions and patient reaction to having a wound, must also be included. The importance of clear understandable documentation to ensure continuity and good communication cannot be stressed enough. This chapter focuses on the assessment and documentation of chronic wounds or those healing by secondary intention, e.g. pressure ulcers, dehisced surgical wounds, pilonidal sinus excision.

Approaches to wound assessment

There are various indices of healing that serve as parameters on which healing can be assessed in wounds healing by secondary intention. Instruments are available that can help us to predict wound development such as the Waterlow Scale (Waterlow 1985) (Figure 5.1) which, when used in conjunction with clinical judgement, can alert professionals to the possibility of tissue breakdown at an early stage.

Methods for classifying wounds abound (e.g. staging (the European Pressure Ulcer Advisory Panel (EPUAP 1999) pressure ulcer staging; Table 5.1)), for measuring wounds (e.g. tracing) and for assessing wound status or the clinical appearance of wounds (e.g. the red, yellow, green and black classification (Table 5.2)).

Other classifications do so by assessment of damage via tissue layer, others by the colour and nature of material occupying a wound bed. These methods are perhaps over-simplifying a very complex situation, with both having disadvantages. Classification by tissue layer assumes knowledge of the anatomy of skin and deeper tissue layers, and an ability to recognize the tissues and differentiate between them. It is difficult to stage a pressure

BUILD/WEIGHT FOR HEIGHT	★	SKIN TYPE VISUAL RISK AREAS	★	SEX AGE	★	SPECIAL RISKS TISSUE MALNUTRITION	★
Average	0	Healthy	0	Female	1	e.g. Terminal cachexia	8
Above average	1	Tissue paper	1	Male	2	Cardiac failure	5
Obese	2	Dry	1	14–49	1	Peripheral vascular disease	5
Below average	3	Oedematous	1	50–64	2	Anaemia	2
		Clammy (temp ↑)	1	65–74	3	Smoking	1
		Discoloured	2	75–80	4		
		Broken/spot	3	81+	5		

CONTINENCE	★	MOBILITY	★	APPETITE	★	NEUROLOGICAL DEFICIT	★
Complete/Catheterized	0	Fully	0	Average	0	e.g. Diabetes, MS, CVA	
Occasionally incontinent	1	Restless/fidgety	1	Poor	1	Motor/sensory	
Cath./incontinent of faeces	2	Apathetic	2	Nasogastric tube/fluids only	2	Paraplegia	4–6
Doubly incontinent	3	Restricted	3	NBM/anorexic	3		
		Inert/traction	4				
		Chairbound	5				

MAJOR SURGERY/TRAUMA	★
Orthopaedic – below waist spinal	5
On table > 2 hours	5

MEDICATION	★
Cycotoxics	4
High-dose steroids	
Anti-inflammatory	

SCORE	10+ AT RISK	15+ HIGH RISK	20+ VERY HIGH RISK

Figure 5.1 The Waterlow Pressure Sore Prevention Treatment Policy. Ring scores in the table and add total. Several scores per category can be used. (Reproduced with permission from Judy Waterlow.)

Table 5.1 EPUAP Pressure Ulcer Classification

Grade	Description
1	Non-blanchable erythema of intact skin; discoloration of the skin, warmth, oedema, induration or hardness may also be used as indicators, particularly on individuals with dark skin
2	Partial thickness skin loss involving epidermis, dermis or both. The ulcer is superficial and presents clinically as an abrasion or blister
3	Full-thickness skin loss involving damage to or necrosis of subcutaneous tissue that may extend down to, but not through, underlying fascia
4	Extensive destruction, tissue necrosis or damage to muscle, bone or supporting structures with or without full-thickness skin loss

EPUAP (1999)

Table 5.2 The clinical appearance of wounds – colour classification (see Plates 4–8)

Colour	Clinical appearance
Black	Necrotic area of hard, dead tissue
Yellow	Slough: dead cells accumulated in exudate
Green	Infected: pus with offensive odour; signs of inflammation
Red	Granulating tissue
Pink	Epithelialization: white/pink tissue

Adapted from Cuzzell (1988)

ulcer, for example, when the wound is filled with necrotic tissue. Classification using thickness says nothing about the condition of the surrounding skin, level of exudate or odour – factors that will strongly influence dressing selection. Colour classification is useful, if only to remind nurses what type of material is present in the wound (Table 5.2). However, when nurses are questioned about what they understand by 'granulation tissue' a large number are unable to answer.

The colour classification has been expanded to include pink and green, with each colour describing the clinical appearance of the wound surface. In spite of criticism that the system is simplistic, it is useful as part of a more comprehensive assessment to provide guidance. The overall aim is to standardize nursing language in relation to wound management to improve documentation and communication.

Wound assessment parameters

Davis et al. (1992) suggest that six aspects must be taken into account when considering the management of a patient with a wound:

1. the site: the range of tissue types involved and the anatomical position of the wound
2. stage: how far the healing processes have progressed
3. cause: the nature of the wound, i.e. burn, trauma, surgery
4. form: the size, shape and state of the wound. Irregularly shaped wounds will be more complicated to dress and heal than open cavity wounds.
5. environment and carer: in home, hospital, self-care or nursed. Consideration must be given to the resources, knowledge and skills available wherever the patient is cared for.
6. health-care system: the organization and delivery of care.

Harding (1996) describes a wound-healing matrix that is intended to provide a basic structure to the decision-making process, not as a rigid and inflexible tool, but as an aid to choosing appropriate care and management. The components of the wound-healing matrix reflect the six aspects listed above (Davis et al. 1992).

The aetiology of the wound

Identification of the aetiology of the wound is vital information required to inform treatment decisions. Reliable information must be obtained from the patient, relatives or carers about the history of the wound using focused questioning. Often it is easy to identify pressure damage from the position of the patient lying in the bed; accurately diagnosing leg ulcers, e.g., is more complex. With advances in technology, there are now several different assessment methods available, both to clarify and/or to confirm the aetiology of the wound, and its extent, which is not always obvious. These technologies will not always be readily available for routine use but nurses should have some knowledge of what is available (Collier 2003):

- Doppler ultrasonography: a method for determining systolic pressure more effectively and more accurately than with a stethoscope; used when calculating the ankle–brachial pressure index (ABPI)
- colour duplex scan (colour flow Doppler ultrasonography): used to provide information on the arterial wall, width of lumen and blood flow
- photoplethysmography (PPG): a non-invasive test using an infrared light source and a transducer light probe to provide a measure of venous reflux and venous filling times (Doughty et al. 2000)

- phlebography: injection of a radio-opaque dye into the lower limb veins to detail the venous system
- sonography, computed tomography (CT) and magnetic resonance imaging (MRI)
- there are several non-invasive, computer-based, assessment systems available commercially which can be used to determine wound dimensions accurately.

The overall appearance of the wound

There is no 'standard' wound; a wound may contain a mixture of tissue which may be necrotic, granulating and part epithelializing depending on the aetiology, condition of the patient and the way it has been managed. Nurses should be able to identify the tissue present in the wound and attempt to estimate the approximate percentage of different tissue present to form a baseline for future comparisons. The mixture of tissue present may complicate the choice of dressing/therapy but the same assessment principles will apply. The clinical appearance of wounds is discussed.

The clinical appearance of the wound

Wounds containing devitalized tissue: the black necrotic or yellow sloughy wound

Local tissue death can be identified from the presence of necrosis and slough in a wound. This can present as black or brown, dehydrated, leathery eschar or scab, or soft, yellow, grey or off-white material adhering to the wound base. Other terms used to describe the presence of dead tissue are dry gangrene, for uninfected necrotic tissue, and wet gangrene, which implies superadded infection, non-viable tissue and devitalized tissue.

Necrosis is the result of tissue losing its blood supply (ischaemia) and therefore the essential nutritive elements and oxygen to the cells. An available vascular supply that is rich in nutrients and oxygen is vital for supporting cell metabolism and without it the cells die. Thomas (1990, 1997b) suggests that slough may be composed of either devitalized tissue or a mixture of fibrin, protein, exudate, leukocytes, giving a creamy yellow colour (Flanagan 2001), and bacteria. There is little known about the constituents of necrotic tissue but it is assumed that it consists of dried blood, exudate and denatured proteins, such as collagen, elastin, fibrin, haemoglobin and other coagulation proteins (Thomas et al. 1999). The aetiology of the injury governs the appearance of devitalized tissue; what is usually seen in the wound is the build-up of dead cells, either dried (necrotic) or moist (slough).

Thomas et al. (1999) found that necrotic tissue has a structure similar to healthy human dermis with scattered areas of disrupted or degraded tissue. This study highlighted the dearth of knowledge in this important area and how further research is needed to aid understanding of the complex processes involved.

As the devitalized tissue dehydrates and shrinks, in black necrotic wounds, Thomas (1997b) suggests that reversal of this process, i.e. re-hydration of devitalized tissue, may alleviate pain. The presence of devitalized tissue in a wound will impede healing by extending the inflammatory phase of healing so its removal is essential (Flanagan 1997a). Necrotic tissue builds up in a wound; when the normal processes fail to cope with the accumulation of excessive amounts of devitalized tissue, the natural process is overwhelmed and inadequate (Ramundo and Wells 2000).

There are several recognizable types of necrosis associated with different origins:

- coagulation caused by ischaemia resulting in tough, black necrosis
- liquefaction in which there are large numbers of white cells resulting in a softer, yellow or white, sloughy appearance
- caseous associated with tissue infection and presents as soft, friable whitish-grey necrosis
- gangrenous which is a combination of coagulation and liquefaction where the blood supply is lost.

The presence of necrotic tissue prevents epidermal cell migration and epithelialization, and slough inhibits the movement of epithelial cells. There are also problems associated with assessing the depth and extent of the wound when it is filled with necrotic tissue – another valid reason for its removal.

Within the wound, necrotic tissue may be tightly bound to the wound base as with black leathery tissue or thick, 'tethered' slough or fine and stringy slough (almost the consistency of chewing gum). Exposing soft, moist slough to the air may cause it to become hard and leathery. Moist wound healing has been advocated since the early 1960s (Winter 1962) as the most efficient method for supporting optimal healing.

Factors influencing necrosis

Tissue death can happen for many reasons; the following are some of the unfavourable conditions for healing.

Extrinsic factors

Mechanical stress

- Pressure: if pressure is exerted at a specific, localized area it may be intense enough to reduce or prevent capillary blood flow to the area leading to hypoxia or ischaemia. If the pressure is relieved, the area may re-perfuse, restoring the blood flow and oxygen to the tissues without long-term detrimental effects. Depending on individual circumstances and the length of time, it is possible that the blood vessels will remain closed and the area will become ischaemic with further destruction at the wound site.
- Shear: shearing forces may be strong enough to separate the dermis from the underlying tissue and destroy the capillaries.
- Friction: recurrent friction causes the outer skin surface to abrade, in time deepening to affect the underlying tissues that house the capillaries. Appropriate patient-handling techniques using approved manual handling aids should be used to prevent damage to the skin and underlying structures.

Intrinsic factors

Changes resulting from the ageing process
Skin fragility and reducing blood supply are key factors in increasing the risk of tissue damage and necrosis. Slower healing occurs as a result of delays in the start of the inflammatory phase, slower cell migration, reconstruction and scar formation, and generalized slower cell metabolism.

General health status
The functional delivery of oxygen and nutrients to the cells can be impaired in several ways: lack of or poor nutritional intake; cardiovascular disease causing reduced delivery of oxygen and nutrients to the cells, e.g. arteriosclerosis, venous insufficiency, peripheral artery disease; diabetes mellitus (with associated atherosclerosis, arteriosclerosis, neuropathy, delayed response to injury and defects in the formation of scar tissue, poor glycaemic control); anaemia (reduced ability to transport oxygen to the cells); and reduction in immune function (necessary for the inflammatory phase of healing and avoidance of infection).

Poor nutrition
Without adequate supplies of the right kind of food (carbohydrates, protein, fats, vitamins, trace elements and fluids) wounds will not heal; they will remain in a state of limbo where no improvement is seen for long periods of time.

Miscellaneous factors

These include: lifestyle factors, such as over-indulgence in alcohol leading to digestive problems, malnourishment, liver damage and anaemia, cigarette smoking (reduces the amount of oxygen delivered to the cells); body build: obesity – poor wound healing, wound dehiscence, poor eating habits, poor vascularization in fatty tissue, poor mobility. Underweight individuals may suffer from inadequate food intake to build up energy stores (Cutting 1994).

All of these factors may influence the wound healing process, resulting in the recurring development of necrotic tissue if not corrected or alleviated in some way.

Autolysis

Autolysis is generally defined as 'the breaking up of living tissues' (Weller 2000) or, more particularly with regard to wounds, the natural degradation of devitalized tissue (Davis et al. 1992) or self-destruction. It is a naturally occurring bodily function achieved by the action of enzymes and macrophages digesting necrotic tissue in the wound bed during the inflammatory phase of healing (Rodeheaver 1994). Natural autolysis is a selective method of débridement because it does not affect healthy tissue. Autolysis can take place only within a moist, vascular environment and is dependent on a fully functioning immune system. The process is artificially enhanced by the application of a moisture-retentive dressing to the necrotic wound to allow proliferation and activity of white blood cells and the production of growth factors (Ramundo and Wells 2000).

Wounds containing granulation tissue

Granulation begins approximately 5 days after injury (Davis et al. 1992) with capillaries (angiogenesis), macrophages and fibroblasts moving into the site of injury. Granulating tissue is mainly composed of a complex mixture of polysaccharides and proteins within a highly vascular collagen network. Macrophages secrete growth factors and chemotactic factors which stimulate the fibroblasts to migrate, multiply and deposit matrix (framework for healing). The new capillary network provides the vehicle for oxygen and nutrients to be delivered to the healing tissues.

Granulation tissue is highly vascular and very fragile as a result of the thin walls of the capillaries (one cell thick) and so must be treated gently. Dry dressings must not be used because they will adhere to the new tissue and cause trauma on removal. Open-weave dressings such as tulle dressings are contraindicated for granulating wounds because the capillaries will grow into the open weave, causing trauma on removal.

Healthy granulating tissue is characteristically granular in appearance, bright red and moist, whereas unhealthy granulating tissue appears pale or unnaturally red, and bleeds spontaneously, or as a result of minor trauma.

Overgranulation

Occasionally wounds overgranulate (granulation tissue that is raised above the area around the wound) for no obvious reason, preventing epithelial cells from migrating to cover the wound. This may be related to a defective inflammatory response or unrelieved mechanical irritation (Morison 1992a, 1992b, Dealey 1994). The traditional treatment with silver nitrate is not recommended (McGrath and Schofield 1990, Morison 1992a, Dealey 1994) because it is corrosive. Currently recommended management consists of changing from an occlusive dressing to a non-occlusive dressing (Young 1995), the application of light pressure to the wound (Harris and Rolstad 1992) or the daily topical application of corticosteroid and antibiotic ointment under medical supervision (Thomas 1990).

Epithelializing wounds

Epithelializing wounds are reaching the final stages of healing when epithelial cells are migrating from the margins of the wound to resurface the wound over the newly formed granulation tissue in a full-thickness wound. In a superficial wound, epithelial cells will also originate and migrate from the site of remnants of hair follicles and sweat glands. Epithelial tissue will be recognized by its silvery, pinky-white appearance. Epithelialization may be disrupted by the presence of foreign material, desiccation, temperature and pH changes, and infection in the wound (Davis et al. 1992).

The key to supporting successful epithelialization is protection of the new tissue with non-adherent dressings that maintain a moist, warm, clean, wound environment and are not changed too frequently.

Exudate

Exudate, otherwise known as wound fluid or wound drainage, is defined as a fluid produced in wounds made up of serum, leukocytes and wound debris. The volume diminishes as healing progresses. Exudate is thought to have bacterial and nutrient properties but it may be infected (Cutting 1997). The production of exudate in a wound at different stages of healing is a naturally occurring phenomenon and a vital component for healing as the blood vessels dilate following haemostasis. This happens as part of the normal inflammatory response to enable white blood cells, in particular, to migrate to the traumatized tissue.

Excess wound exudate can cause major problems for both patients and their carers such as soiling of clothes, dislodging of dressings leading to increased infection risk and social embarrassment. Exudate management is possibly one of the most difficult challenges facing nurses in practice in spite of the wide range of management options available.

There is a wide range of absorbent dressings available in varying presentations – ribbon, rope, cavity filler, flat foam dressings, alginates, hydrofibre dressings and various super-absorbent dressings. However, in wounds with exceedingly high levels of exudate other options may be more appropriate, e.g. vacuum-assisted therapy or wound drainage appliances. Vacuum-assisted closure therapy is discussed in Chapter 8.

Black (1995) recommends that wound drainage appliances should be used when drainage is in excess of 100 ml/24 h and that the following factors are considered before choosing an appliance:

- the wound size: most easily accessible wound drainage bags are available in a limited range of sizes from 7.6 cm × 7.6 cm to 10 cm × 23 cm and 21 cm × 21 cm
- the type of wound: postoperative dehisced wound, infected wound or spontaneous fistula
- the type and amount of output or exudate (Pringle 1995): if excessive a drainable bag is preferable
- individual patient needs: long term or short term, for an immobile or mobile patient, with or without access to a porthole for attending to dressing changes
- the shape of the wound must also be considered, because there appears to be a dearth of appliances suitable for circular wounds more than 10 cm × 10 cm
- the relationship of a fistula to other anatomical features (Pringle 1995)
- the condition of the surrounding skin
- the presence or absence of sepsis (Pringle 1995).

Odour

Most wounds do not have an offensive odour so when the wound suddenly becomes malodorous the reason is probably colonization, infection or the presence of devitalized tissue or even a soiled dressing. Malodour can be very distressing for the patient, relatives and carers. It can result in loss of appetite, isolation, relationship problems and depression.

There are difficulties quantifying and describing malodour, as an individual's perception of smell is very subjective. Haughton and Young (1995) attempted to devise a method for quantifying odour through the use of an odour assessment scoring tool shown in Table 5.3.

Table 5.3 Odour assessment scoring tool

Score	Assessment
Strong	Odour is evident on entering the room (6–10 feet or 2–3 metres from the patient) with the dressing intact
Moderate	Odour is evident on entering the room (6–10 feet or 2–3 metres from the patient with the dressing removed
Slight	Odour is evident at close proximity to the patient when the dressing is removed
No odour	No odour is evident, even at the patient's bedside with the dressing removed

From Haughton and Young (1995)

Certain infecting organisms can be identified by their distinctive appearance and aromas, e.g. the fluorescent greenish colour seen on dressings from wounds infected with *Pseudomonas* species has the characteristic odour of *Pseudomonas*. The odour has been described as 'musty'. Wounds infected with staphylococci emit a distinctive putrid smell that is difficult to forget. Several odour-absorbing dressings, some containing silver, are available with the newer silver dressings having the propensity to attract bacteria away from the wound surface, thus reducing the odour.

The nurse is in the ideal position to provide the necessary support and reassurance. Systemic treatment may be with antibiotics if wound infection is responsible for the malodour. If there is necrotic tissue in the wound, this should be removed. Dressings may need to be changed more frequently; occlusive dressings that contain exudate and odour-absorbing dressings may be appropriate. Deodorizers only mask the odour. Larval therapy, sugar paste and honey have been demonstrated to be useful in controlling odour.

Care of the skin around the wound

The skin surrounding a chronic wound is likely to be subjected to trauma from frequent dressing changes and exudate. Care of the surrounding skin must not be forgotten when treating the wound. Trauma must be avoided at all cost, particularly where the skin is paper thin and fragile. Dermatitis or allergies to the dressing or tape may be evident as erythema or blistering. Inadequate dressing absorbency or inappropriate choice of dressing may lead to maceration of surrounding skin, resulting in extension of the original wound and skin erosion. Proactive treatment of the surrounding skin with a barrier film or cream (Cavilon) is required to prevent maceration and excoriation around chronic wounds.

There may be a build-up of dead skin cells around a wound, especially on the feet and legs, because dressings do not allow for normal bathing and the natural removal of dead skin. Regular application of emollients is essential for the skin of patients with leg ulcers to prevent dry, flaky, uncomfortable skin and further skin breakdown under bandaging.

Setting and communicating treatment objectives

Following assessment of the patient, identification of the cause of the wound and correction, if possible, of causative factors, the wound parameters are assessed and documented. This procedure is not a one-off, but must be repeated by the nurse at each dressing change and any changes observed in and around the wound recorded. Wound assessment documentation must complement patient assessment data, e.g. it should be clear from the documentation what has been done in the case of pressure damage to relieve or reduce pressure, whether compression has been used over the dressing for a venous leg ulcer, so that the interventions can be evaluated holistically. Wound assessment charts are ideal tools on which wound assessment data may be recorded. Key assessment parameters are listed on the wound assessment chart and include classification, clinical appearance, exudate, odour, dimensions, pain and the condition of surrounding skin. The use of wound assessment charts is discussed in more detail in Chapter 6.

Recognition of the kind of tissue present in the wound will guide product selection. Wound healing is delayed by the presence of slough or necrotic tissue in a wound (Dealey 1994); its presence will encourage the growth of bacteria, rendering it high risk for becoming infected. Efforts should be directed towards removing necrotic tissue using the most suitable method. Granulating and epithelializing wounds need protection from cold, trauma and too frequent dressing changes.

Conclusion

Before the application of a dressing to any wound, certain principles must be acknowledged and adhered to. These include a thorough patient assessment to identify the factors that have precipitated the chronic wound.

After patient assessment, attempts must be made to correct any of those factors that will respond to correction in order to prevent the risk of recurrence or worsening of the wound. Wound assessment is a complex process that requires wide-ranging knowledge of the healing process, wound management and wound management products. The primary aims of local wound management are to protect the individual from further physiological damage and progress through to uninterrupted healing.

Student exercises

- Construct a list of questions you would ask a patient with a wound.
- Examine your reactions to having maggots applied to your wound.
- Find out whether there is a local wound management formulary and obtain a copy.
- Which members of the multidisciplinary team could be involved in planning care for patients with high levels of exudate?
- Conduct a brief audit of wound management documentation in your clinical area.

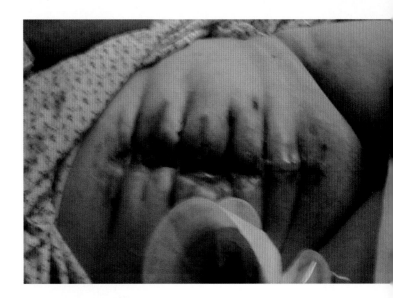

Plate 1 Dehisced abdominal wound due to underlying malignancy.

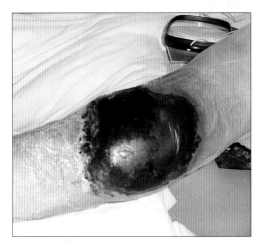

Plate 2 Haematoma.

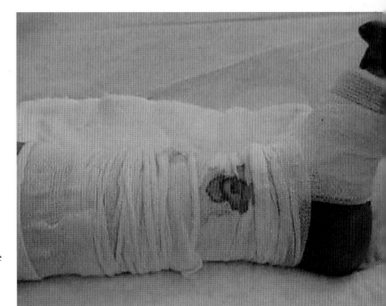

Plate 3 An example of poor bandaging.

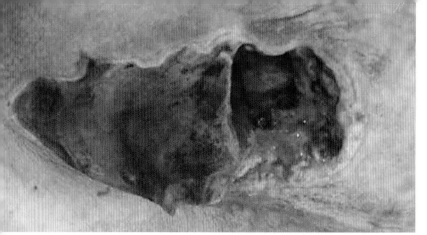

Plate 4 Necrotic pressure ulcer.

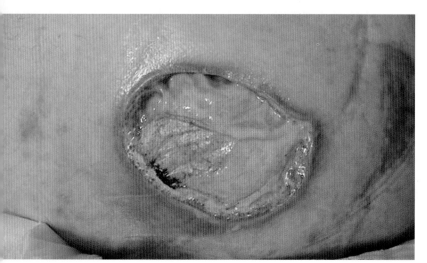

Plate 5 Sloughy pressure ulcer.

Plate 6 Infected leg (cellulitis).

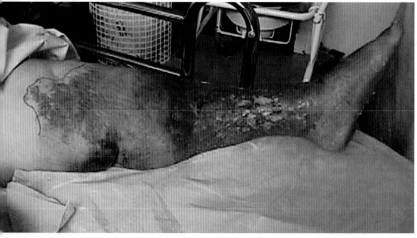

CHAPTER SIX

Documenting wound care

Communicating: preventing misunderstandings

Record keeping is a fundamental part of nursing practice, one that should help the care process; it is not an optional extra and failure to keep such records may be judged to be negligent practice. The Nursing and Midwifery Council (NMC) revised the United Kingdom Central Council (UKCC 2004) *Guidelines for Records and Record Keeping* in 2002. This document gives clear guidance on the standard of documentation expected of a first-level nurse. The NMC also published a *Guide for Students of Nursing and Midwifery* in 2002 outlining good practice. Although students are not professionally accountable to the NMC for the consequences of their actions, they may still be called to account by their university or the law. The guidance given particularly relates to accepting appropriate responsibility (within the limits of preparation), patient confidentiality and complaints. With regard to documentation, students should always have any entries countersigned by a registered nurse.

Good record keeping is a reflection of the standard of an individual's professional practice and a mark of the skilled and safe practitioner; the model chosen should be a product of local consultation and agreement (UKCC 2004). Therefore, comprehensive nursing documentation must complement patient and wound assessment data to aid consistency of care and communication between staff carrying out dressing changes for patients with open wounds. Clinical records are the main source of data and evidence used for dealing with complaints, claims and clinical incident investigations (Pennels 2001). They should at least be available, accurate, easily identifiable, legible, chronological, comprehensive and complete. The practitioner should be aware of the potential audience who may have access to patient records from the patient to a local MP, the police, the Commission for Health Improvement, Professional Conduct Committee, coroner, ombudsman, Audit Commission and solicitors, to name a few.

The legal requirements of charting and recording wound care data

Documentation of care has become synonymous with care itself:

No documentation = No care.

Failure to provide care and/or good documentation and the nurse is deemed an unprofessional practitioner. Assessment of the patient and the wound should be carried out in a methodical manner (Dealey 2000, p. 205). As a minimum, health-care documentation should be the following:

- Accurate: true, objective; a reflection of what should happen or what has happened, or shows concrete evidence of the use of the nursing process.
- Relevant: the patient's history, nursing assessment, problems or concerns, care plans, interventions, a diary of what happened and reference to audit or evaluation of care must be included. Transfer or discharge information should appear as early as possible with evidence of continuity of care. Wound management plans, dressings/therapies should be clearly documented.
- Complete: all pertinent points over the spectrum of nursing care and records should be completed as soon as possible after the delivery of care.
- Concise: records should be written succinctly and precisely; economy with words and short sentences should be the normal practice.
- Timely: the exact timing of an event is important to the accuracy and relevance of treatments or adverse events.
- Legible: common sense prevails here – if a record cannot be read and understood this could contribute to poor care or even negligence. Poor handwriting, spelling, unnatural order of events, obscure abbreviations and the use of inappropriate words are the main causes of illegibility. Nurses may be asked to defend what they have written in court: statistically the records of nurses, midwives and health visitors are poor. At NMC professional conduct hearings, health-care records are used as evidence of accuracy of events surrounding a case, because they are more reliable than a nurse's recollection of the event.
- Written and signed by a responsible registered practitioner who has cared for the patient.

Nurses should be alert and not become complacent about documentation. A record of untoward events must be kept as well as incident reports completed and submitted to risk management in the event of a pressure ulcer occurring.

Documenting wound care

The way wound care is documented varies enormously between health-care organizations. It has only been over recent years that nurses have realized that standardization of documentation and multidisciplinary access to patient records is beneficial. In the field of pressure ulcer prevention and wound management, it is normally nurses who take the lead when decisions are made about treatment. Several reasons for this may explain why doctors take a back seat (Dealey 2000):

- Doctors do not receive the relevant education in their training.
- Pressure ulcers have traditionally been the 'fault' of nurses.
- There is less written about the topic in medical journals than in nursing journals.
- Nurses tend to have more knowledge and skill in relation to products/therapies and their application.
- There is historical conflict between nurses and doctors about what is the best dressing/cleansing solution for the patient's wound.

Along with the advent of clinical nurse specialists for tissue viability came a valuable educational resource for all members of the multidisciplinary team and for the patient, relatives and carers. A major part of the role is teaching about prevention and management of wounds and how to produce documentation that meets local and national standards. The introduction of, for example, wound assessment charts will focus the attention of the nurse towards completeness, accuracy and good written communication.

Wound assessment charts

In the quest for encouraging comprehensive documentation several wound assessment charts have been devised (Morison 1988, Carroll and Johnson 1991, Miller and Powell 1995, Bale and Morison 1997, Dealey 2000) which list the wound parameters that should be assessed and documented each time a wound is re-dressed (Figure 6.1). These variously include: wound classification, clinical appearance, exudate odour, dimensions, pain and the condition of surrounding skin. Others include parameters such as signs of infection and information about whether wound swabs have been taken, and previous dressing use or allergies to wound care products, which is useful information for the clinician. The aim of recording assessment data is to aid consistency of care and communication between staff carrying out dressing changes for patients with open wounds.

Patient ID label	Ward: Date: Wound type: Location: Duration: Special aids in use: Frequency of dressing change:
Allergies?	
Previous dressings:	Swab sent: Yes No Date swab sent:

Weekly tracing of the wound and measurement, complete chart and record in nursing evaluation.

Assessment	Date	Date	Date	Date	Date	Date
Clinical appearance: a. Sloughy b. Necrotic c. Granulating d. Epithelializing						
Exudate a. Colour b. Amount c. Type						
Odour a. Offensive b. Not offensive						
Pain a. Location b. Type c. At dressing change only d. Pain score 1–5						
Wound margin a. Red b. Eczema c. Swollen						
Infection a. More than two signs of inflammation b. Send swab to confirm						
Dressing planned a. Hydrogel b. Hydrocolloid c. Alginate d. Hydrofibre e. Foam f. Other therapy						

Figure 6.1 An example of an open wound assessment chart.

The Department of Health (DoH) has recently reinforced the NMC's emphasis on the importance of good record keeping by including it as one of the 'Essence of Care' patient-focused benchmarks for health-care practitioners (DoH 2001b).

Documenting information about the wound

The following observations should be documented (Culley 2001):

- wound type and location: chronic or acute, aetiology; body maps are useful to site wounds
- wound size, shape and its margin: measurement, tracing and description of the margin
- appearance and colour: using approved classification systems
- nature and amount of discharge/exudates: not easy to measure but estimates can be made by describing the number of dressing changes required and their frequency
- signs of clinical infection: heat, redness, pain, oedema, pus, loss of function
- where possible, wound mapping should be encouraged as part of the wound assessment.

The following is an example of appropriate initial assessment documentation about a patient admitted with a wound:

Admitted from home with a sloughy sacral pressure ulcer approximately 10 cm × 10 cm with extensive undermining. The surrounding skin is macerated as a result of excessive exudate. Previous dressings used at home include foam cavity filler and adhesive foam dressing. No obvious signs of clinical infection.

General medical condition poor, dehydrated, malnourished and unresponsive.

This would be followed by documentation regarding the management of the wound and the patient. If the wound has a mixed appearance, there should be an attempt to estimate the percentage of, for example, slough and granulation tissue for future reference. Changes to the plan of care should be clearly recorded, dated and signed, and progress evaluated.

Measuring and charting wound dimensions

There is no simple, accurate method for measuring progress in wound healing. One relatively reliable and easy method is to measure the dimensions of the wound with a ruler at the widest and longest points.

Measurement is then recorded in centimetres or inches, and a tracing can be made using a clear, sterile, plastic sheet or one of the measuring grids provided by manufacturers of certain wound care products (i.e. hydrocolloid and film dressings), or a double thickness of the sterile, clear, plastic packaging may be used. The wound edges must, however, be clearly identifiable to obtain an accurate tracing. After tracing, the soiled sheet is discarded and a copy placed in the patient's case notes. The area of the wound can be calculated using graph paper.

All tracings and measurements must be clearly labelled (indelible ink must be used) left and right, top and bottom, with the patient's name, part of the body, unit number and the date of the tracing. Tracing should be done at regular intervals, e.g. weekly or fortnightly to assess progress; however, the accuracy of using such measurements should be considered (Anthony 1993). Measurements must be supplemented in the documentation or on the tracing by a description of the type of tissue in the wound (Pudner 1997). More sophisticated methods, not widely available for use in routine wound care practice, that produce three-dimensional images of wounds are discussed by Vowden (1995).

Alternative methods of recording wound dimensions: photographs and digital images

Tissue viability nurses routinely photograph wounds using either Polaroid cameras or digital cameras. Telemedicine relies on the provision of a clear image in electronic form being transmitted for remote assessment at another centre by other specialists (Newton et al. 2000).

Serial photographs for measuring wound healing progress provide useful records and teaching aids but are of limited value for measuring wound healing progress (Bale and Morison 1997). A disposable tape measure with the date and patient's initials should be placed alongside the wound so that future comparisons can be made. Observations can easily be made of the condition of the skin surrounding the wound as it changes during treatment. Patients often like to see photographs of their wounds if they are physically unable to see the actual wound, e.g. if the wound is located on the back.

In most trusts, the permission of the consultant as well as informed patient consent are required, often in writing, before a wound is photographed. Great care must be taken to ensure that the patient cannot be identified from the photograph. The purpose for which the photograph is being taken, which may be for monitoring progress or educational reasons, should be explained to the patient before the use of a camera. Even with modern technology, it is sometimes difficult to obtain a good quality image. Bellamy (1995) advises consideration of the choice of equipment, materials, lighting, background, focal distance and angle when taking photographs. Even with permission, the patient should never be subjected to prolonged exposure or inconvenience for the sake of photographing a wound.

Concerns have been raised among tissue viability nurses about the possibility of tampering with digital images using specialized software, but no legal guidance has been offered to date. This is an issue linked to professional accountability and public trust in practitioners.

Other methods of measurement, not readily available to the average practitioner include planimetry, wound moulds, foam dressings, three-dimensional measurements and fluid instillation. An advantage of using these methods is that they give an indication of wound depth.

Additional information

The following additional information should be documented for those patients with pressure ulcers: identified risk factors, when the damage was first observed, re-positioning schedules and length of time sitting in a chair (NICE 2001), the grade of ulcer, preventive measures, type of mattress (when supplied) and cushion (type and when supplied), clinical management and evaluation of care. Without this kind of information, it is difficult to track the occurrence of pressure damage for audit purposes and in case of complaint.

Nelson (2000) provides useful guidance on describing the anatomical location of wounds and on taking photographs that will enhance written documentation. Of course, all of this is worthless and a waste of time if nurses do not have the knowledge either to assess and treat wounds, or to read and follow the prescribed care.

Conclusion

Good quality documentation is essential, not just in the event of complaint or litigation but also primarily to direct appropriate day-to-day patient care.

Student exercises

- What are your responsibilities regarding documenting care?
- Examine the wound care documentation in your organization and compare it with what is accepted best practice.

CHAPTER SEVEN

Basic tools for providing the optimal wound healing environment

Wound management

A dressing is described as a covering on a wound that is intended to promote healing and provide protection from further injury (Dealey 2000). This is a rather narrow view of what has become a very complex, sophisticated, expensive and demanding field of care. The term 'wound management products' is probably more appropriate and refers to the many products currently available for dressing wounds and applying to wounds for the purposes of cleansing, débriding, absorbing exudate and providing an environment that will allow the wound to heal at the optimal rate.

It must be clear from the outset, however, that there is no dressing available that can compensate for an uncorrected pathological condition (Bolton et al. 1990); dressings do no more than facilitate wound healing by providing the optimal local environment for healing to proceed. Tissue repair will occur only in the presence of adequate oxygen and nutrients and in the absence of factors that interfere with, or deter, healing. So, those factors that will impede healing, such as poor vascular supply or compromised nutritional status, need to be identified and corrected, if possible (Benbow 2001). Patient assessment factors may include cardiovascular and pulmonary function, nutrition and fluid status, and metabolic conditions, e.g. diabetes, steroids, smoking, immune status and advancing age (Bryant 1987, Flanagan 1989, Doughty 1992, Morison 1992a, Cutting 1994, Dealey 2000).

Moist wound healing

Winter (1962) can be said to have pioneered the work into the development of modern wound management products. Using an animal model he demonstrated that epidermal repair happened twice as fast on wounds covered with a vapour-permeable film dressing compared with those left to scab over. In later studies, other benefits were realized. Enhancement of the natural process of autolysis (the breaking down of devitalized tissue) was observed within a moist environment (Friedman and Su 1982) and local wound pain control was achieved using this method (Friedman and Su 1982, Eaglstein 1985, Alvarez et al. 1989).

Many modern wound management products provide the desired effective environment for healing: moist, clean and warm. Moisture, however, can cause maceration of the surrounding skin; it is often that fine balance between wet and dry at the wound surface that is difficult to achieve. This is where accurate and timely wound assessment is vital.

Product types

Morgan (1997) categorizes wound management products by their performance profiles:

- passive products: cotton wool, gauze, lint and tulles are used to cover, insulate and protect; some are absorbent
- interactive products: films, foams, hydrogels, hydrocolloids, alginates and other polymers; these provide the optimal healing environment
- bioactive products: intervene in the healing process by optimizing what we believe to be the ideal conditions for healing. Alginates, hydrocolloids and hydrogels are both interactive and bioactive. Dressings have now been developed that incorporate growth factors and other environment-modifying elements.

The unit cost of modern wound management products could be viewed as high compared with traditional dressings but this must be weighed against cost-effectiveness relating to a product that promotes fast wound healing and improves the patient's quality of life (Hampton 1999). Many of the modern wound management products require infrequent changes and therefore interfere less with the patient's lifestyle and wound healing.

Following patient and wound assessment, the key to effective wound management is knowledge of the capabilities of particular dressings and how they should be used in individual circumstances. Much is demanded by nurses of dressings as outlined by Turner (1982) in his seven criteria for the optimum dressing:

1. to maintain high humidity at the wound/dressing interface
2. to remove excess exudate
3. to allow gaseous exchange
4. to provide thermal insulation
5. to be impermeable to bacteria
6. to be free of particles and toxic wound contaminants
7. to allow removal without causing trauma to the wound.

Several more criteria could be added to this, e.g. to prevent damage to the surrounding skin, to be acceptable to the patient and to be inexpensive to budget holders.

Wound cleansing

The aims of wound cleansing are to remove any foreign matter such as gravel or soil, and any loose surface debris such as necrotic material and the remnants of the previous dressing (Dealey 2000). However, Thomlinson (1987) demonstrated that the action of cleansing did not reduce the number of bacteria, but merely redistributed them. Traditionally, antiseptics such as EUSOL and chlorhexidine have been used to cleanse wounds, but Russell et al. (1982) proved that antiseptics would need to be in contact with the wound for 20 minutes before they destroyed bacteria.

There are various disadvantages associated with the use of antiseptics for wound cleansing; some general ones are (Lineaweaver et al. 1985):

- They are rapidly inactivated when they come into contact with body fluids or organic material.
- They can cause irritation and sensitivity.
- They are cytotoxic to new cells.

The controversy surrounding the use of antiseptics in chronic wound care continues (Gilchrist 1999). Hohn et al. (1977) found that wound fluid contained cells and chemicals that work to combat infection, leading to the belief that frequent removal of exudate and cleansing is unnecessary and undesirable. To summarize, there is little to recommend the use of antiseptics for routine wound cleansing, although some have limited use for the initial cleansing of traumatic wounds. Dealey (2000) recommends 0.9% saline as the only completely safe cleansing agent and this is the treatment of choice for cleansing most wounds. Saline suitable for irrigating wounds is supplied in sachets, plastic tubes and aerosols.

Many surgical wounds require no cleaning (Pudner 1997). Irrigation at a pressure of 8 lb/in^2 (psi) (Pudner 1997) with isotonic saline solution at room temperature or warmed in warm water (Flanagan 1997b) is recommended as the gentlest and most effective method for removing debris, foreign material and bacteria. However, nurses must be aware of the danger of splash-back to the eyes when irrigating and take appropriate action to protect themselves (Oliver 1997). Bucknole (1996) recommended bathing or showering as suitable methods for cleansing sacral, perineal wounds and leg ulcers, and tap water is increasingly being used in the community and accident and emergency (A&E) departments (Hollinworth and Kingston 1998).

Methods of débridement

Débridement, defined as the removal of devitalized tissue and foreign matter from a wound (Cutting 1996), can be achieved in several ways:

- Surgical excision: should be carried out only by a suitably qualified, competent clinician. Surgical débridement is not always appropriate or without complications (Ballard and Baxter 2001) (see Figure 7.1).
- The application of soaks or wet packs: this method is very time-consuming and may cause maceration of the wound and surrounding skin (Thomas 1997a). Trauma and pain may be caused by the dressings drying out.
- Hydrogel dressings: to aid autolysis, which is the natural degradation of devitalized tissue by macrophage activity and proteolytic enzymes released at the time of cell death. The enzymes digest cell contents and produce tissue necrosis (Davis et al. 1992). Hydrogels support hydrolysis and work by preventing loss of water vapour from the wound surface and adding fluid to devitalized tissue hydrogels. Their action aids the separation and removal of non-viable tissue from viable tissue. Hydrogels should be covered with a secondary dressing which prevents moisture loss from the gel by evaporation or by absorption into the outer dressing; film dressings are recommended.
- Hydrocolloid dressings: to aid autolysis (as above) by maintaining a moist wound environment.

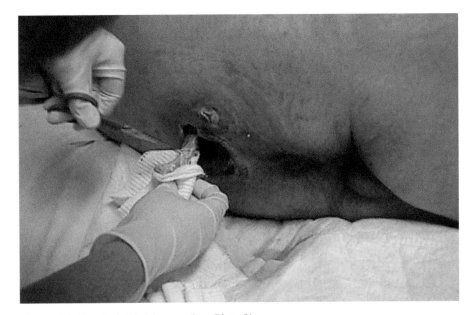

Figure 7.1 Surgical débridement (see Plate 9).

- Alginate and hydrofibre dressings: to absorb exudate in wet wounds and aid autolysis of soft slough when the alginate has gelled.
- Larval therapy: for the rapid removal of devitalized tissue (Thomas et al. 1996). Larval therapy is gaining in popularity because of its rapid, cost-effective and effective way of removing necrotic tissue. There are aesthetic issues concerning the application of live creatures associated with flies to a wound, but it is rare that patients refuse to consider larval therapy.

Other less commonly used débriding agents include crab collagenase (Vowden and Vowden 1999), honey (Cooper and Molan 1999), sugar paste (Topham 2000) and papaya (Starley et al. 1999).

Flanagan (1997b) lists the following factors that will influence the choice of débridement method, but warns that desloughing should be carried out with caution to prevent unnecessary trauma (Flanagan and Graham 2001):

- The type of injury and potential contamination: foreign bodies need to be removed to prevent infection and potential 'tattooing' of the skin.
- The wound aetiology, e.g. diabetic ulcers containing devitalized tissue are high risk for infection so early débridement is usually indicated.
- The size of the wound: large necrotic areas are best dealt with by surgical débridement whereas smaller areas can be débrided using interactive dressings. Larval therapy (otherwise known as maggot therapy or biosurgery) will effectively remove devitalized tissue through the production of powerful enzymes that break down and remove dead tissue, thus promoting granulation tissue formation.
- The extent of tissue damage and type of tissue involved: care must be taken when wounds contain structures such as tendon, muscle or bone. These wounds should be surgically débrided only by a trained and competent clinician. Some wound management products, e.g. hydrocolloids, are contraindicated for use in wounds where bone, muscle or tendon is exposed because they may cause further dehydration of the tissue.
- The amount of exudate: in wounds with large volumes of exudate the priority will be to absorb the exudate with an alginate or hydrofibre dressing which, when it has gelled, is capable of débriding moist slough (Flanagan 1997b).
- Vacuum-assisted closure (VAC) may be appropriate for high exudate wounds where it is thought the reduction in localized oedema leads to increased blood flow and improved healing (Collier 1997). Hard necrotic areas will require the application of hydrogels (with vapour-permeable film secondary dressings) or hydrocolloids as secondary dressings to facilitate autolysis.
- Time available: the availability of appropriately qualified clinicians to

débride may be a problem in the community, necessitating a longer period for débriding the wound using more conservative methods.

- User skill, knowledge base and professional accountability: the range of 'me-too' (i.e. similar dressings to what are already available) wound management products increases weekly, which makes it difficult for practitioners to make appropriate choices. Wound care formularies have gone some way towards rationalizing dressing choice but nurses do not always have the appropriate knowledge of the properties and potential uses of different products to ensure that appropriate choices are made (Flanagan 1999).
- Cost-effectiveness: the initial/unit costs of VAC therapy or larval therapy may appear high but the effectiveness, reduction in healing times and reduced dressing frequency of such options outweigh the costs.
- The care environment (hospital or community): certain therapies are not available in the community as a result of funding restrictions. This may mean that the patient is admitted to hospital or the costs are borne by the acute trust for treatment in the community.
- The patient's wishes: patients must be kept fully informed about the advantages and possible disadvantages of proposed therapies so that they are in a position to consent as appropriate.

Following débridement, the aim will be to support the process of healing by providing optimal conditions at the wound surface: moist, clean and warm (Winter 1962).

Why dress wounds?

Thomas (1997a) summarizes the main reasons for health-care professionals deciding to apply a dressing as follows:

- to produce rapid and cosmetically acceptable healing
- to remove or contain odour
- to reduce pain
- to prevent or combat infection
- to contain exudate
- to cause minimum distress or disturbance to the patient
- to hide or cover a wound for cosmetic reasons
- a combination of two or more of the above.

From a patient's perspective the considerations for having a dressing in place may be different from those of the practitioner. Patients with chronic wounds have probably been through a large range of available dressings and will have strong views about what suits them. Other factors that will influence product choice may include continence status, known sensitivity, fragile skin, bathing frequency, social circumstances, wound aetiology and the patient's ability or desire to comply with the treatment.

From the practitioner's perspective, an awareness of the unit cost of individual dressings is required because many of the modern products are substantially more expensive than traditional dressings (Thomas 1997a). Arrangements for the supply of dressing products can be confusing because in some acute trusts a range of dressings will be stored and supplied from the on-site hospital pharmacy and via the supplies department. There may be problems associated with ordering from a regional stores warehouse because this may take up to 3–4 days. In such cases, ward stocks may have to be depleted in order that patients can take sufficient dressings home with them.

Wound management product grouping by properties and actions

The categorization of wound management products is becoming more complicated as new, different and combined dressings appear on the market. This section categorizes the more common types of dressing by their properties. The main groups of dressing that provide the optimum wound healing environment are films, hydrogels, hydrocolloids, alginates, foams and hydrofibre dressings. Dressings from each group will, in the right circumstances, assist healing and débridement of wounds.

Primary wound dressings

Low-adherent dressings, e.g. Release, N-A Ultra, can be regarded as low adherent rather than non-adherent and should be used only for wounds with low exudate; they need to be covered with tape or a secondary dressing. Low adherent dressings can be used as carriers for hydrogels on sloughy or necrotic wounds covered with a semi-permeable film dressing. N-A Ultra is recommended when adherence to the wound is a potential problem (Thomas 1997a).

An example of a medicated, low-adherent dressing, Inadine, is impregnated with povidone–iodine and is indicated for shallow, open, clinically infected wounds, e.g. minor burns, superficial skin loss injuries, or diabetic or ischaemic ulcers. Inadine should be avoided in patients with sensitivity to iodine or povidone–iodine and with thyroid disorders. Exudate levels dictate the frequency of dressing change. If a large volume of exudate is being produced the dressing will probably need a daily change. Therapeutic antibacterial levels are unlikely after 2 days (Thomas 1997a). Adherence may be a problem, in which case the dressing can be loosened with warmed saline.

Film dressings

These products, e.g. Tegaderm, Op-site, usually consist of a thin polyurethane membrane coated with a layer of acrylic adhesive (usually hypoallergenic – Thomas 1997a). They are permeable to water vapour and oxygen but impermeable to bacteria. The wound-healing environment therefore remains clean, warm and moist, with the moisture preventing the development of a scab on the wound surface. Films as primary dressings are suitable only for non-clinically infected, shallow, low-exudate wounds, e.g. pressure ulcers, minor burns, lacerations and abrasions. Pain caused by the exposure of nerve endings is reduced within this environment. Film products may also be useful to reduce friction and for protection of vulnerable skin. As secondary dressings, they are useful to cover hydrogels, alginates and hydrofibre products to prevent them from drying out. Because they are transparent, it is possible to observe the wound through the dressing. Many film products have novel presentations that aid their application.

Manufacturer's recommendations for application, removal and wear time should be followed. When applying film dressings they should not be stretched so that the skin wrinkles after application because this may cause blistering. When removing a film dressing, an edge should be carefully lifted and the body of the dressing stretched parallel to the skin in the direction of hair growth, supporting the rest of the dressing with the other hand. In between stretches, relax and then stretch again to break down the adhesive. This will prevent trauma to the surrounding skin and wound, and reduce pain. There are also special techniques to apply films to awkward places such as the heel or elbow by cutting and applying the film in strips or shaping it to fit around fingers and hands comfortably. Film dressings can be left in place for up to 7 days depending on the level of exudate and retention ability.

Amorphous hydrogels

Hydrogels, e.g. Intrasite, Intrasite Conformable, Nu-Gel, GranuGel, Purilon Gel, consist mainly of water (about 80–94%), polymer, humectant and preservative. They have a propensity for donating fluid when placed in contact with a wound. The main indications are for sloughy, dry, necrotic wounds such as pressure ulcers, leg ulcers, extravasation injuries and surgical wounds, and work by re-hydrating dead tissue. Hydrogels can, however, be

used effectively throughout healing on low-exudate, granulating and epithelializing wounds. Hydrogels do not absorb fluid, so they are not
recommended for wet wounds. A secondary dressing is always needed.
Ideally, they should be covered with a semi-permeable film dressing to prevent the gel drying out and to support autolytic débridement. The
frequency of dressing change will depend on the state of the wound and
effectiveness of de-sloughing. On exuding wounds, this may be daily whereas on drier wounds the hydrogel may be left for up to 3 days (Thomas 1994).

Hydrocolloids

Hydrocolloids, e.g. Duoderm, Cutinova Hydro, Comfeel Plus, Tegasorb,
are interactive dressings that consist of cellulose, gelatines and pectins,
with a backing made of polyurethane film or foam. They are self-adhesive
and so do not need a secondary dressing. Hydrocolloids are indicated for
wounds with low-to-medium exudate, such as pressure ulcers, leg ulcers,
minor burns and traumatic wounds, from which they can absorb and hold
exudate in the hydrocolloid matrix. Hydrocolloids are completely impermeable to water vapour and therefore support re-hydration and autolytic
débridement of necrotic and sloughy wounds. Bathing or showering
is possible without removing the dressing because of its waterproof
properties. Pain is reduced when the dressing is in place and removal is
usually atraumatic if the dressing is removed by pulling back on itself, like
removing a sticking plaster. Application and adhesion are facilitated by
warming the dressing between the hands before application and when in
place. The hypoxic environment created by hydrocolloids is said to encourage angiogenesis (Cherry and Ryan 1985).

A problem common to many adhesive dressings is rolling of the edges,
particularly when applied to the sacrum as the patient moves about. A small
amount of talcum powder applied to the sticky edges may prevent the edge
catching on the clothes or bedclothes. A general rule is that hydrocolloids
should not be left in place for more than 7 days (Thomas 1994).

Hydrocolloids are available in many different presentations for both flat
wounds and cavity wounds. A newer adaptation is Aquacel, which is a highly absorbent, flat sheet dressing or ribbon made of hydrocolloid fibres,
which forms a thick conformable gel when it absorbs exudate (Flanagan
1997b). Cutinova Cavity and Aquacel are both suitable for heavy-to-moder-
ately exuding wounds (Dealey 2000).

Alginates

These dressings, e.g. Kaltostat, Sorbsan, Tegagen, SeaSorb, are derived
from different types of seaweed and are suitable for moderate-to-heavily

exuding wounds. The fibrous dressing gels when it absorbs exudate, producing an appropriate environment for healing. Kaltostat also has a product licence for use as a haemostat. They are indicated for highly exuding pressure ulcers, leg ulcers and fungating wounds, and are most useful for exuding cavity wounds. Alginates need a secondary dressing to contain moisture and aid autolysis. Dressings are easily removed in one piece with a gloved finger or forceps. Dressing change intervals will depend on the exudate levels, but alginate dressings should not be left in place for longer than 7 days in a non-infected wound (Thomas 1994).

Polyurethane Foam dressings

Foam dressings, e.g. Allevyn, Lyofoam Extra, Tielle, Cavi-Care (formerly Silastic foam), are made of polyurethane or silicone, are presented as either flat dressings or fillers for cavity wounds, and can be adhesive or non-adhesive. The wound side is constructed so that it takes up large amounts of blood and exudate by capillary action into or across the dressing. Some foam dressings have an outer vapour-permeable polyurethane film backing. The purpose of the vapour-permeable backing is to allow the passage of moisture out of the dressing, to reduce build-up with associated skin and wound maceration underneath the dressing.

Adherent foam dressings are indicated for moderate- to high-exudate wounds and provide an effective barrier to bacteria. As a result of the construction of the contact layer of the dressing, it will not stick to the surface of the wound. Foams will not provide any therapeutic benefit for dry necrotic wounds. Non-adherent foams should be held in place with thin strips of adhesive tape along the edges or a retaining bandage. On a clean, non-infected wound, the dressings can be left in place for 4–5 days (Thomas 1994). Cavi-Care is a foam product that must be mixed with a catalyst before being poured into the cavity wound, where it moulds to the shape of the wound. Foam sheet dressings are frequently used as secondary dressings over alginates and hydrofibre dressings. The many and varied shapes and sizes available attempt to meet the demands of all types and locations of wounds, e.g. Allevyn sacral dressing, Allevyn heel dressing.

Miscellaneous dressings: charcoal dressings, skin protectants, antibacterial dressings, tulle dressings

Charcoal dressings

Charcoal dressings, e.g. Actisorb Silver 2000, CarboFLEX, Carbonet, Lyofoam C, are constructed of activated charcoal cloth and work by absorbing the chemicals released from malodorous wounds. The inclusion of silver in Actisorb Silver 2000 is said to attract bacteria into the dressing away from the wound. Antibacterial dressings include Arglaes, Flamazine (silver sulfadiazine) and Metrotop gel (metronidazole gel).

Arglaes is a semi-permeable film dressing containing silver ions recommended for wounds infected with methicillin-resistant *Staphylococcus aureus* and other bacteria. Flamazine, a cream containing 1% silver sulfadiazine, is effective against a wide range of bacteria used for burns and leg ulceration. Metrotop gel contains metronidazole (0.8%) and is a very effective deodorizer in pressure ulcers, fungating wounds and other lesions infected with anaerobic organisms. For clinically infected wounds, the appropriate antibiotic cover would be necessary. Metrotop gel would normally be used in conjunction with systemic metronidazole for best effect (Bale 1997). Dressings containing silver are discussed in Chapter 9.

Skin protectants

Maceration and damage to the skin surrounding a wound is a major problem associated with chronic and infected wounds, and the frequency of re-dressing. Cavilon has, over the last few years, become a popular and effective addition to many formularies for protecting skin before the application of adhesive dressings as well as in the treatment of excoriated, macerated skin caused by incontinence, oral dribbling and leaking stomas. Cavilon, supplied as either a spray or a swab, should be applied to the affected skin and left to dry for 30 seconds. One application should last 2–3 days according to the level of moisture present. Cavilon Cream is also now available.

Tulle dressings

Tulle dressings are less popular than in the past; as knowledge develops and technology advances, the faults of traditional methods become clear. There are two main problems associated with tulle dressings when used as primary dressings: granulation tissue grows into the open weave of the tulle and is torn away on dressing removal, and they dry out quickly. These products have been largely superseded by modern wound management products.

Matching the wound type to the wound management product

The necrotic wound

Necrotic tissue consists of dead cells in exudate that has dried and must be removed from a wound, mainly to reduce the risk of infection, but also to facilitate healing. The aim of treatment will be to re-hydrate dead tissue to help it to separate from viable tissue in the wound. The most commonly used dressing is the hydrogel because it contains 94% water, which, when in contact with the wound, will be taken up by the necrotic tissue. As the necrotic tissue softens it also separates, leaving a clean wound bed ready for granulation tissue to form. A secondary dressing must be used to prevent the gel drying out, so film, hydrocolloid or foam dressings will be appropriate.

The sloughy wound

Slough also consists of dead cells in exudate but it is moister than necrotic tissue. If, however, the wound is infected it may be heavily exuding; hydrogel products will make the wound even wetter. A hydrofibre or alginate dressing may be more suitable for use, because it will absorb and gel. The gel maintains moisture at the dressing–wound interface to support de-sloughing by autolysis if covered by an occlusive or semi-occlusive secondary dressing. Combination dressings of hydrogel and alginate/hydrofibre should never, therefore, be necessary.

Larval therapy is an effective alternative for de-sloughing and débriding sloughy and necrotic wounds quickly and efficiently.

The granulating wound

The choice of dressing for any wound will depend on the site, shape, depth, level of exudate, material occupying the wound, level of knowledge of the practitioner and, to some degree, patient preference and previous experience, e.g. allergies or sensitivity to particular dressings.

In the case of granulating wounds, the aim will be to maintain a moist, warm, clean wound surface and to avoid maceration and desiccation. For cavity wounds with medium-to-high exudate there are many cavity fillers available such as alginates and hydrofibre dressings to a varied range of foam dressings, all of which are absorbent. A choice between those with adherent borders and those without will be made based on the location of the wound and the condition of the surrounding skin.

Care must be exercised when using Cavi-Care not to allow it to flow into sinuses or cavities where the extent of the wound is unknown. A piece of foam may break off and lead to a foreign body reaction or the formation of an abscess (Thomas 1997a). For flatter drier wounds, there are dressings such as hydrocolloid wafers, and flat foam adhesive and non-adhesive dressings.

The epithelializing wound

The traditional low-cost treatment for epithelializing wounds has been tulle products, e.g. paraffin gauze, Jelonet. These are gradually being super-seded by dressings such as hydrocolloids, semi-permeable film dressings, silicone dressings (Mepitel) and wound contact layers (Tegapore, Urgotul) which do not dry out, adhere to the wound or cause pain and trauma on removal. Some can be left in place for up to 14 days. Paraffin gauze dress-ings impregnated with antibiotics or antimicrobial agents should not be used topically because there is the constant risk of skin sensitivity and, on a wider scale, bacterial resistance (Thomas 1997a). The best advice for treating an epithelializing wound is to apply a non-adherent dressing and leave it for as long as it will remain in place.

For detailed discussion about the management of malodorous and infected wounds the reader is referred to Collier (2000), Kiernan (1997) and Gilchrist and Morison (1992).

Practical issues

Practical issues, important to both the nurse and the patient, when select-ing dressings, include ease of application and removal, conformability and comfort when in place. These factors can make a big difference when attempting to gain patient compliance and nursing compliance to, e.g. a local formulary.

Patients with hand injuries, unfortunately, are still treated with fabric dressings and bandages and told not to get the dressing wet. This is com-pletely impractical advice to give to a young mother with babies to look after and unnecessary when there is such a wide range of modern water-resistant dressings available to choose from.

Wound infection and dressings

The choice of wound dressing will be determined by the need to control the symptoms (Gilchrist and Morison 1992). The presence of clinical infection, if suspected, should be confirmed by the microbiologist and sys-temic antibiotics prescribed. Modern wound management products can be used in conjunction with antibiotics but the usually high exudate levels in infected wounds will increase the frequency of dressing change. It is, how-ever, advisable to check an infected wound daily while exudate levels are high and malodour is a problem. Certain dressings such as DuoDERM, Granuflex, Tegaderm and Tegasorb are not recommended for use on clinically infected wounds (Surgical Materials Testing Laboratory Dressing Data Cards: www.smtl.co.uk). If in doubt about using a particular dressing on a clinically infected wound, contact the manufacturer (manufacturers' helplines are available) or local representative. As the infection resolves, exudate will decrease and dressings may then be left in place for longer periods.

Conclusion

There is no one dressing for each wound; rather there is a variety of dressings that the nurse can use to provide the best conditions for healing (Doughty 1992). The nurse must, however, take the time to learn about different wound types and how their characteristics change, available dressings and their indications, properties and guidelines for use so that the correct match can be made for each individual circumstance. The range of products increases daily and now, with the advent of more advanced technologies, it becomes ever more difficult to justify and defend the choices made. Decisions need to be made about whether technologies such as vacuum-assisted therapy, hyperbaric oxygen, larval therapy or even alternative and complementary therapies become part of the nursing wound management repertoire in view of cost and available evidence of efficacy.

Student exercises

- From where would you obtain information about dressings?
- On what basis would you choose to use a hydrogel dressing?
- What advice would you give a patient leaving hospital/clinic with a dressing in place?

CHAPTER EIGHT

Modern wound management technologies

Alternative therapies for managing wounds

Wound management is becoming a more complex and sophisticated area of nursing practice. The number of patients with chronic wounds appears to be increasing in line with current demographic changes, causing more time to be spent assessing, treating and evaluating the effects of novel treatment modalities. This is a fascinating time for nurses with a particular interest in wound management, with the development of many and varied therapy options being added to their repertoire for treating wounds. There are still, however, problems associated with correct and appropriate use of conventional wound management products that have been in use over the last 10–15 years, so change will necessarily be slow. Nurses in general still have much to learn about moist wound healing, dressing choice, available products, their composition and modes of action, indications and contraindications, wear time and expected outcomes. In spite of this they are faced with innovations that, it is claimed by manufacturers, can potentially improve the rate of wound healing, be cost-effective and convenient to use. What must never be forgotten is the fact that products and devices do not heal wounds; healing will always require correction of the underlying factors that militate against healing, i.e. ensuring the patient is in the best condition for healing to happen. Nurses have a professional and moral obligation to keep their practice up to date and provide the best standards of care for patients (UKCC 1996). Justification for the use of some of the new therapies is difficult, so any ideas of demonstrating a sound evidence base can and must be challenged.

The focus so far has been on modern wound management products that are now regarded as conventional approaches for supporting wound healing. More frequently, practitioners are managing wounds with what may still be considered innovative therapies such as vacuum-assisted closure, larval therapy, laser therapy and treatments that manipulate the properties of the healing wound.

Vacuum-assisted closure (vacuum therapy, vacuum sealing or topical negative pressure therapy)

The application of vacuum-assisted closure (VAC) negative pressure to a wound stimulates the blood supply, removes exudate and stimulates the production of granulation tissue. The advantages of using VAC therapy are accelerated healing time, reduced bacterial colonization, reduced odour and the convenience of exudate being drawn away from the wound leaving a neat dressing which allows the patient to be more mobile. Disadvantages include the patient being attached to a machine and VAC therapy can be difficult to apply and is expensive (Collier 1997, McCallon et al. 2000).

VAC therapy consists of a machine that applies controlled levels of either intermittent or continuous negative pressure to a wound. The system creates a hypoxic environment in which aerobic bacteria cannot survive and 'pulls' blood that is rich in growth factors and macrophages into a relatively uncontaminated area (Hampton 1999). Therapy has been shown to accelerate débridement, promote angiogenesis, and remove slough and loose necrotic material in many different wound types. The dressing consists of black open-cell foam for cavity wounds and white, flat, small-cell foam for flat wounds. The foam is cut and tailored to the shape of the wound ensuring a snug contact with all surfaces of the wound. A perforated, tubular, plastic wound drain is placed over the foam and the whole area is sealed with a film dressing to make it airtight. The tubing is connected to a canister that fits into the machine creating a closed drainage system. There are two types of machine, a mains-operated system (ATS) with a 300-ml canister and a smaller, portable, battery-powered system with a 50-ml capacity canister for the more mobile patient at home with lower exudate levels.

Visual and audible alarms warn when the dressing seal is broken, the canister is full or the system is tipped or not on a level surface. A negative pressure of 125 mmHg is recommended as optimal for most wounds with lower pressures applied for skin grafts and leg ulcers. When the dressing is sealed in place and the pump is switched on the negative pressure causes the foam dressing to be sucked inwards and go hard, drawing the wound edges in with it.

The underlying principle of VAC therapy is not a new idea; surgeons have employed various suction drainage methods for years. The difference with the VAC system is that suction is effected uniformly across the surface of the whole wound. When in place and working, a partial vacuum is formed within the wound, reducing its volume and facilitating the removal of fluid (Thomas 2001).

Clinical indications for VAC therapy

These are across a wide range of wounds:

- chronic non-healing wounds such as pressure ulcers (Deva et al. 1997, Fabian et al. 2000)
- venous and arterial ulcers and diabetic ulcers (Hartnett 1998)
- dehisced surgical wounds (Tang et al. 2000a, 2000b)
- traumatic wounds (Fleishman et al. 1993)
- flaps, grafts and burns (Mullner et al. 1997, Banwell 1999)
- infected wounds (Tang et al. 2000a, 2000b). Collier (1997) reported a reduction in wound colonization by 1000 times in 4 days in infected wounds treated with VAC therapy.

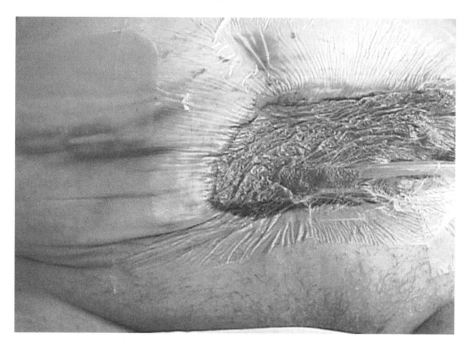

Figure 8.1 VAC therapy (see Plate 10).

VAC therapy is particularly useful for large, heavily exuding wounds that are difficult to manage with conventional products. The potential for clinical infection is reduced as exudate is removed (Collier 1997). VAC therapy is contraindicated in the presence of active bleeding, fistulae of unknown origin, opening into a body cavity, vulnerable body organs, malignancy, dry, necrotic tissue and untreated osteomyelitis. Care must be exercised when patients are receiving anticoagulant therapy.

Possible complications to VAC therapy include allergic reactions to the drape, pressure necrosis from the tubing, pain, growth of granulation tissue into the foam dressing, fistula formation and an increase in blood flow to neoplasms. There are always disadvantages associated with new therapies. VAC therapy is not inexpensive: rental of the therapy unit is currently £30–39, dressings between £18 and £20, and canisters between £11 and £13. The company recommend that dressings be changed every 48 hours and the canister changed and discarded either when full or at a maximum of 4 days, and the dressing technique is complicated. If the dressing is left for more than 48 hours granulation tissue will grow into the foam causing firm adherence, pain and bleeding. This can be prevented by lining the wound cavity with a small pore, non-adherent dressing (Urgotul, Mepitel) or an N-A Ultra dressing. Alternatively, a measure of hydrogel dressing can be applied to the wound bed. In practice, VAC therapy can be cost-effective, very effective and convenient, removes excess exudate and odour, and is well accepted by patients and clinicians in spite of limited scientific proof of its usefulness.

Larval therapy

Larval therapy (biosurgery, maggot therapy) is not a new concept; it has been around for centuries. Sterile larvae, from *Lucilia sericata* (green-bottle), are bred and supplied by the Biosurgical Research Unit (Bridgend). When supplied for use each larva is approximately 2 mm long; after therapy they increase in size to about 8–10 mm. One treatment comprises approximately 300 live larvae, which are supplied in a sterile container. The number required to treat a wound will be determined by the size of the wound and the amount of necrotic tissue contained within it (Thomas et al. 2001). Their development, and therefore efficacy, can be adversely affected by residues of hydrogel dressing containing propylene glycol in the wound (Thomas and Andrews 1999). The maggots are instrumental in removing slough and bacteria, deodorizing wounds and stimulating the production of granulation tissue (Thomas et al. 1996) efficiently and in a very short time.

Clinical indications for larval therapy

- sloughy or necrotic wounds, particularly those that have proved resistant to autolytic débridement attempts, such as pressure ulcers (Sherman et al. 1995)
- leg ulcers (Sherman et al. 1996)
- ischaemic and diabetic ulcers (Thomas et al. 1996)
- infected wounds including those infected with methicillin-resistant strains of *Staphylococcus aureus* (Chaffrey 1997, Thomas et al. 1999).

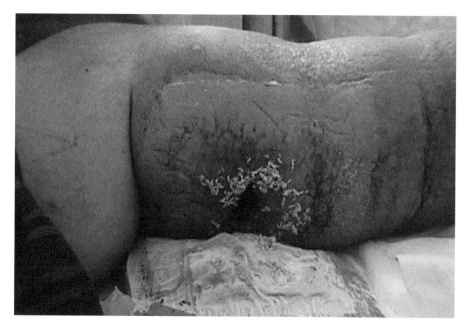

Figure 8.2 Larval therapy to calf wound (see Plate 11).

The mode of action of the larvae is to break down and liquefy necrotic tissue by secreting proteolytic enzymes, causing the wound to bio-débride, kill bacteria by ingestion, digestion and antibacterial secretions (Pavillard and Wright 1957), and the stimulation of healthy granulation tissue (Prete 1997). The precise mechanism is unknown but larval therapy is very effective in reducing odour and exudate in infected wounds. Healthy human tissue is unaffected by the action of the larvae (Thomas et al. 1998).

Application technique

Explicit directions for application of the larvae are supplied with a fine-bore nylon net to contain the larvae within the wound. The dressing technique comprises: protecting the surrounding skin with a hydrocolloid dressing up to the wound edge, placing the larvae into the wound (after loosening them from the container with saline) and covering them with the mesh secured around the edges with waterproof tape (Sleek) over the hydrocolloid. Moistened gauze should be placed over the mesh to ensure that the larvae do not dry out. If there are high exudate levels padding may be lightly applied over the mesh, secured around the edges and changed as required – the area must not be occluded. For difficult-to-dress hand and foot wounds, mesh sleeves or boots can be requested and applied in a similar manner.

The larvae are left for 3 days when they can be removed with gloved fingers, if necessary, or rinsed from the wound with saline and disposed of as clinical waste. There is usually a marked improvement in the wound even after a single application, but if, on further wound assessment, additional applications are considered necessary, they may be applied in the same way.

Disadvantages of larval therapy relate to the aesthetics and cost. A 3-day single treatment (one container) will cost approximately £50 plus dressings, but, in most cases, will considerably reduce the length of time taken to débride the wound. Any proposal for using larval therapy must be fully explained to patients, so that they can give informed consent, and to their relatives. In practice, it is more often nurses rather than patients who will object to the idea of larval therapy. Nurses must be comfortable with the idea and competent to apply the dressing. In the experience of the author, patients have been more than happy to try alternative methods for shortening their hospital stay and healing their wound more quickly. Although a dramatic improvement in wound débridement is often witnessed after a single treatment, the mode of action is not fully understood (Thomas et al. 1998).

The use of silver in wound management

There has been a recent resurgence of interest in the use of silver for its antibacterial properties in wound care as a result of increasing problems associated with antibiotic resistance (White 2001). Silver sulfadiazine has been used to treat burns and grafted areas for many years for its effectiveness against *Pseudomonas aeruginosa* and haemolytic streptococci (Fakhry et al. 1995). Silver nitrate has traditionally been used to treat overgranulation of wounds.

Several wound management products containing silver are commercially available as hydrofibre, foam, hydrocolloid, film and composite dressings.

White (2001) suggests the following as characteristics of the ideal silver dressing:

- delivers silver in a sustained therapeutic way into the wound
- combined antimicrobial effect and capacity to absorb exudate
- has an odour-control function
- easy to apply and comfortable for the patient
- cost-effective.

The mode of action of silver-containing dressings is primarily to release continuously small amounts of antimicrobial silver into the wound to inhibit the growth of bacteria. The potential value of silver-containing dressings is currently attracting a lot of interest and they could have an increasing role in managing wound infection effectively.

Hyperbaric oxygen therapy

Hyperbaric oxygen therapy (HBOT) involves the delivery of 100% oxygen inside a treatment chamber at a pressure greater than that at sea level. One hundred per cent oxygen is breathed intermittently while the pressure of the treatment chamber is increased. At a pressure of 3 atmospheres (303 kPa), dissolved oxygen in plasma is sufficient to supply tissue requirements without drawing from oxygen bound to haemoglobin. The therapy grew from problems experienced by divers exposed to high pressures. It is widely accepted as standard treatment for decompression illness, gas gangrene and gas and air embolism, and used as an alternative adjunct treatment for a wider range of conditions:

- diabetic wounds including diabetic gangrene and diabetic foot ulcers
- necrotizing fasciitis and Fournier's gangrene
- post-radiation therapy tissue damage
- preparation for surgery in previously irradiated tissue (Department of Health or DoH 2003).

HBOT encourages wound repair in two ways in the hypoxic and/or infected wound: first, by wound hyperoxia satisfying the need for increased aerobic metabolism, supporting increased requirements for the healing processes and, second, by increased nitric oxide (free radical) production by the wound which regulates the microcirculation and endothelial cells (Boykin 2002).

Chronic wounds caused by underlying peripheral vascular disease, diabetes, radiation necrosis, soft tissue infections, and some osteomyelitic and traumatic wounds are suitable for HBOT. Contraindications include recent or significant ear or sinus surgery, chemotherapy, seizures, claustrophobia and febrile disorders (Boykin 2002).

Medicinal leeches

In the nineteenth century, leeches were used for 'blood letting' – a cure for anything from headaches to gout. The use of leeches has declined as modern medicines and surgical techniques have evolved, but they are still used today to relieve venous congestion and severe swelling in plastic and reconstructive surgery. Their beneficial actions are thought to be caused by chemicals secreted in their saliva which can prevent clumping of platelets and interrupt blood coagulation, so helping to restore blood circulation to grafted tissues and re-attached appendages.

Medicinal leeches are applied as a last resort; patients may be hesitant but receptive to the idea when it may mean the difference between salvaging and losing a part of the body. When therapy begins it continues until new blood vessel connections form around the affected tissues so they can re-establish perfusion. The number used will vary according to the tissue response. The therapy is painless partly because the nerves are already amputated; the leeches' saliva contains an anaesthetic and anti-clotting agent that keeps the blood flowing freely. They can devour up to five times their body weight within 30 minutes, after which they will drop off. They should be disposed of as clinical waste after use.

Honey

The use of honey is also currently enjoying a revival for its antibacterial properties when modern therapies have failed. Honey has been applied to wounds since about AD 50 and has recently been shown to be effective against over 60 species of bacteria, including aerobes, anaerobes, Gram-positive organisms, Gram-negative organisms and resistant strains of *Streptococcus pyogenes* and *aureus*. Other beneficial effects include antifungal (Molan 2001), deodorizing, anti-inflammatory and débriding actions. The therapeutic effect of honey is produced by low concentrations of slow-release hydrogen peroxide found naturally in the honey and its high osmolarity, which inhibits antibacterial action (Molan 2001). Honey has been used for a range of wound types such as burns, pressure ulcers, venous leg ulcers, pilonidal sinuses (Betts and Molan 2001) and infected wounds that are unresponsive to conventional treatments (Efem 1988).

Honey is commercially available in sheet or gel form which, depending on the exudate level, is applied to the wound and covered with an absorbent or film dressing. The frequency of dressing change will depend on how rapidly the honey is diluted by exudate. Honey is also available in some countries combined with an alginate in the dressing; it can be inserted into cavity wounds or injected into sinuses because it is water soluble and may be rinsed away (Molan 2001).

A possible disadvantage associated with the use of honey may be the need for frequent dressing changes as a result of its dilution by exudate. It has, however, been shown to be non-irritant (Subrahmanyam 1996), soothing (Subrahmanyam 1993) and pain free on application (McInerney 1990), with no adverse side effects reported (Ndayisaba et al. 1993). Further research in the use of honey as an effective wound dressing is planned in the UK.

Wound drainage bags

Wound drainage bags are designed to cope with varying amounts of liquid or semi-solid matter. Wound drainage management may be required for postoperative draining wounds, fistulae, sinuses, dehisced wounds or heavily infected wounds.

The fundamental practical considerations relate to maintaining the integrity of the surrounding skin and controlling the effluent (Black 1995) for any wound that is heavily exuding to the point where wet dressings are in contact with areas of skin. In the case of fistulae, if not controlled and depending on the point of origin of the fistula, corrosive gastrointestinal effluent from the wound can rapidly cause problems of skin excoriation, leading to pain, soreness, itching, infection and ulceration. This, in turn, will affect the patient's mood and sense of well-being even further. Without doubt, high-quality general clinical patient support is vital because often they are very ill people, probably suffering from the effects of dehydration, malnutrition, infection, illness and surgery. Large wounds and fistulae will take many weeks to heal, i.e. if they are going to heal; sometimes nursing care can only hope to contain the problem. This situation causes the patient and family much anxiety and frustration with frequent dressings, soiling of nightclothes and bedclothes, and embarrassment when nurses have to re-dress the wounds or change the drainage bag.

Few, if any, modern absorbent dressings can cope with the effluent from a fistula as a result of the continuous production and sometimes changing consistency. Prone nursing to encourage drainage has been attempted in the past (Patey et al. 1946), but there are still the problems of wet dressings in contact with the wound and surrounding skin.

Skin barrier preparations should be used to protect skin from the damaging effects of effluent, e.g. Cavilon, or wafer dressings, e.g. Stomahesive. Ideally, skin barriers should be applied before excoriation occurs because skin excoriation will hinder adherence of the wound drainage appliance and potentially reduce wear time.

Black (1995) recommends that wound drainage appliances should be used when drainage is in excess of 100 ml/24 h and that the following factors are considered before choosing an appliance:

- the wound size
- the type of wound: postoperative dehisced wound, infected wound or spontaneous fistula
- the type and amount of output or exudate (Pringle 1995): if excessive a drainable bag is preferable
- individual patient needs: long term or short term, for an immobile or mobile patient, with or without access porthole for attending to dressing changes

- the shape of the wound must also be considered, because there appears to be a dearth of appliances suitable for circular wounds larger than 10 cm × 10 cm
- the relationship of a fistula to other anatomical features (Pringle 1995).
- the condition of the surrounding skin
- the presence or absence of sepsis (Pringle 1995).

There is a wide range of devices designed to cope with various sizes of wounds, those that need to be dressed or irrigated several times a day, those in awkward places and where effluent is semi-solid.

The obvious advantages associated with a well-fitting, correctly applied, closed drainage system relate to patient comfort and confidence. Odours and exudate or effluent from the wound are contained and managed appropriately. This will minimize leakage on to bedclothes and night-clothes which can be very distressing to patients and relatives. Careful skin preparation and protection of the surrounding area will make all the difference when wear time and, therefore, cost-effectiveness are considered. The correct application of wound drainage bags requires skill, patience and knowledge of the material components of the system. Ensuring a flat surface by the use of filler pastes facilitates the application and subsequent adherence to the skin. Newer skin barriers such as Cavilon have properties that overcome the problems of heat and perspiration as well as corrosive effluent, and can be used under hydrocolloid dressings placed around the wound to protect the skin.

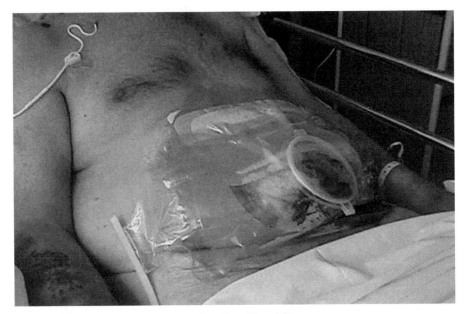

Figure 8.3 Wound drainage bag in place (see Plate 12).

Applying wound drainage bags

The wound should be measured with the patient lying flat; a template can be made and used for cutting out to a size slightly larger than the wound. The skin is cleansed and the surrounding skin dried; any crevices should be filled as necessary or the area covered with a thin hydrocolloid. Stomahesive paste may be applied to the edges of the wound. It is essential to take time to apply the appliance carefully to ensure a good seal as it is pressed into place. Replaceable filters that should be changed every 24–36 hours are available with some appliances. Those appliances with portholes are useful if there is a wound that needs dressing, for inspection or for wound irrigation. It is desirable for a wound management appliance to remain in place for 4–7 days, depending on the wound and provided that the skin has been treated appropriately and it is not being corroded by effluent. It should be noted that not all wound management appliances are sterile.

The successful management of patients with fistulae and heavily exuding wounds presents many challenges to nurses (Dealey 2000), patients and their carers. The principles of fistula management are suggested as follows:

- to fit and maintain a suitable, comfortable, leak- and odour-proof appliance
- to protect the skin around the fistula to prevent excoriation and discomfort
- to ensure collection of output to assess loss so that correct replacements can be given
- to facilitate trust and understanding between the patient and the multidisciplinary team, creating the optimum environment for recovery to take place (Elcoat 1986).

Electrical stimulation therapy

Theories associated with the effects of electrical currents on healing wounds date back to the 1600s when gold foil applied to wounds was found to promote healing and prevent scarring (Robertson 1925, cited by Broussard et al. 2000). Becker (1961) hypothesized that the body maintains an electrical current within itself that is responsible for healing – a theory that has provided a basis for a developing body of knowledge that relates to the role of electrical stimulation in wound healing.

There are four main types of electrical stimulation: low voltage, continuous direct current, low or high voltage-pulsed current and pulsed electromagnetic energy delivered at varying rates. The charge is applied via electrodes placed over saline-soaked gauze on or around the wound for

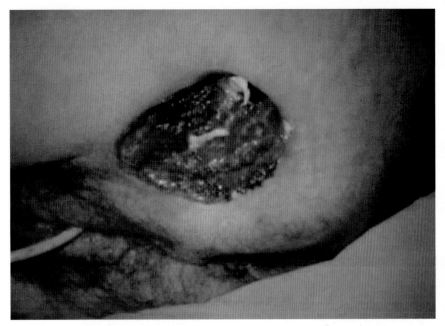

Plate 7 Granulating pressure ulcer.

Plate 8 Epithelialising leg wound following haematoma.

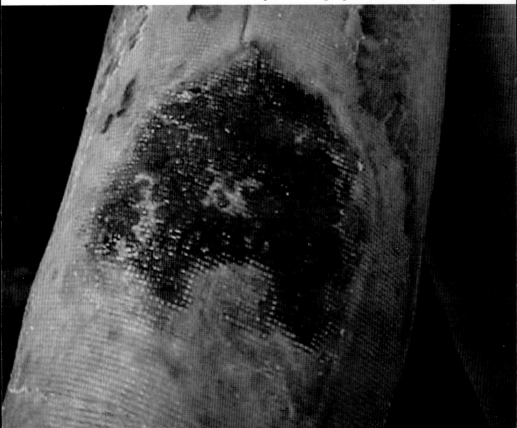

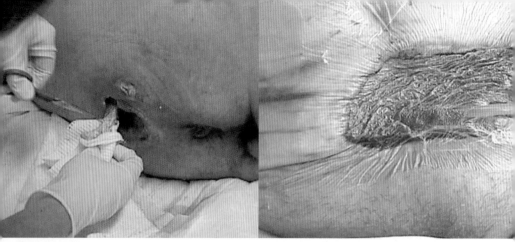

Plate 9 Surgical débridement.

Plate 10 Vacuum Assisted Therapy.

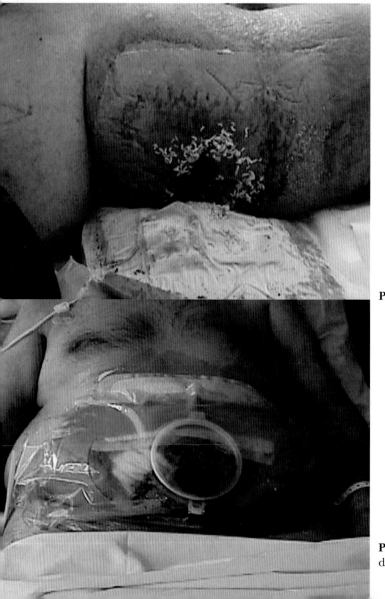

Plate 11 Larval therapy.

Plate 12 Wound drainage bag in place.

between 30 minutes and 4 hours per treatment once or twice daily until healing occurs (Broussard et al. 2000). Foulds and Barker (1983) suggest that electrical stimulation may work by mimicking the natural currents of the injury either re-starting or accelerating the wound-healing process. Improved blood flow (Hecker et al. 1985), bacteriostatic effects (Fakhri and Amin 1987), débridement and stimulatory effects on cells (Alvarez et al. 1983) have been demonstrated during electrical stimulation.

Electrical stimulation has been evaluated on a range of chronic wound types, including pressure ulcers, diabetic ulcers, venous and arterial ulcers and acute traumatic wounds (Broussard et al. 2000). Only one randomized double-masked study of pulsed electromagnetic energy for healing pressure ulcers, in spinal cord-injured patients (Salzberg et al. 1995), has been carried out. This study demonstrated a significantly shorter healing time.

Disadvantages associated with the use of electrical stimulation are the training requirements, the complexity of the therapy, the expense of, and access to, the machine, the time required for setting up therapy and the limited evidence available for its efficacy.

Ultrasound therapy

The basic mechanism of healing by ultrasonography is the stimulation of cell activity in the wound, along the path of the ultrasound beam, acting as a stimulus that the cells transduce into electrical and thermal energy (Dyson and Lyder 2001). Ultrasonography can reduce the length of the inflammatory phase of healing so that the wound enters the proliferative phase more rapidly, assisting the body to heal itself (Dyson 1995). These actions are dependent on the presence of intrinsic factors that support healing in the patient. Chronic wounds need to be débrided so that they are in the acute inflammatory phase of healing before therapy. Pain and oedema reduction have been reported following ultrasound therapy (Sussman and Dyson 1998).

Laser therapy

Laser (light amplification by the stimulated emission of radiation) therapy is directly applied around the wound area or to a wound covered with a transparent dressing if the skin is damaged. The energy, applied through a probe, is said to trigger cell activity, particularly macrophages, in the wound area which accelerates healing (Dyson and Lyder 2001). Low-intensity laser therapy is a popular modality usually applied to chronic wounds by experienced physiotherapists. For nurses, therefore, therapy is limited to when it can be provided by physiotherapists. The initial outlay for machinery is costly and evidence of efficacy scanty.

Cullum et al. (2001) found that there is generally insufficient reliable evidence to draw conclusions about the contribution of laser therapy, therapeutic ultrasonography, electrotherapy and electromagnetic therapy to chronic wound healing. There are also practical problems associated with regular attendance and therapy time to apply the treatment.

Long-term use of wound contact dressings

A number of dressings are now available that are designed as primary wound contact layers or membranes that remain in place until the wound is healed. They are vapour permeable, non-adherent, maintain a moist environment and allow exudate to pass through into the secondary dressings, which will be replaced when exudate strikes through or according to the manufacturer's recommendations. The wound contact layer may be left in place for 1–2 weeks or until the wound has healed. Some long-term use dressings have a similar, small-pore, open-weave design to tulle dressings but, because they contain silicone gel and their manufacture is based on a particular technology, they do not stick to the wound. These dressings will adhere only to dry skin (and the clinician's gloves) and will not allow the ingrowth of granulation tissue with subsequent pain and trauma on removal (Mepitel). Tegapore consists of chemically inert hypoallergenic polyamide net and acts in a similar fashion to Mepitel.

Tegapore and Mepitel can be left in place for up to 14 days on clean exuding wounds. Urgotul is another option, with a similar design, but consisting of lipido-colloid technology, which is proving to be an excellent non-adherent dressing over time in place on the wound (Benbow and Iosson 2004). The difficulty is persuading nurses and doctors to leave them in place for the required length of time to make them cost-effective; the main advantage is absence of trauma and pain on removal.

Tissue culture

Tissue culture is the grafting of laboratory-grown sheets of human cells (cultured keratinocytes) on to a granulating wound instead of a skin graft. Tissue taken from the patient has been shown to be more effective than that taken from a donor (Kakibuchi et al. 1996). Although cultured keratinocytes have been used successfully for burn wounds and leg ulcers, the technique needs further investigation and refinement.

Tissue engineering

This goes a step further than tissue culture in that human dermal fibroblasts are cultured on a biosynthetic scaffold (Dealey 2000) for application to the open granulating wound. An ideal environment for healing is reproduced by the living tissue replacement, provided that the wound is infection free. Apligraft and Dermagraft are examples of engineered tissue. Dermagraft is produced from the cells of circumcised babies' foreskins. Most of the research of these products has been conducted on patients with diabetic ulcers and venous leg ulcers with encouraging results (Falanga et al. 1998, Grey et al. 1998a). To date, the initial cost of tissue-engineered products has precluded their wider use, but, if healing is achieved and/or healing times reduced significantly, they become cost-effective. Another product, Oasis, is currently being evaluated. This product is derived from the small intestine of the pig and has been successfully used in the treatment of wounds in dogs, cats, rabbits, monkeys and horses. It provides an absorbable template for the ingrowth of new tissue in wound care and after surgery.

Wound environment-modifying therapies

Growth factors are proteins used for cellular communication (Greenhalgh 1996) and, in particular, to stimulate cell proliferation throughout the process of healing. To date over 30 growth factors have been identified (Morgan 1997) that either cause cell replication or stimulate the movement of cells. The next stage of research is to work out how they can be used topically. It has been suggested that growth factors may be more effective in defective healing to trigger repair than to accelerate healing in normal tissue (Arnold 1996); little is known about the effect of growth factors in chronic wound healing. Although the technology is not new, the cost of growth factors is very high (Dealey 2000); research is, however, improving insight and understanding of how wounds heal and other physiological processes such as fetal development, ageing and cancer.

Products that can regulate the biological events associated with wound healing have been developed that stimulate the body to facilitate the action of intrinsic growth factors (Promogran) and enrich the wound environment to accelerate angiogenesis, thus reducing the time to healing. Promogran is said to 'rebalance and modulate the pathological wound environment in chronic wounds' (Promogran: literature of Johnson & Johnson, 2002) by protecting growth factors, providing the wound bed is clear of necrotic tissue and not infected. Hyalofil is indicated for difficult-to-heal wounds such as the various recalcitrant ulcerated wounds of the lower limbs described as clinical experiences in manufacturers' literature. There is anecdotal evidence of increased inflammation, granulation and better quality tissue repair with this product.

Conclusion

Tissue repair is extremely complex and often unpredictable, relying on the controlled response to trauma and the intrinsic ability of the body to heal. There are no easy options or blanket treatments as each wound and patient is unique. No therapy, no matter how simple it appears, should be undertaken without indepth knowledge of its potential for benefiting the patient as well as possible adverse reactions. Clinicians need evidence of clinical efficacy supported by education relating to the constituents, application, indications and contraindications before they embark on any new therapy.

Wound assessment must be underpinned by a thorough understanding of the physiology of the skin as well as the delicate process of tissue repair (Flanagan 2003). Nurses have a professional responsibility to stay as up to date as possible, constantly building on basic knowledge to enable informed and logical approaches to managing patients with wounds. Custom and practice and personal preferences have no place in modern patient management; expenditure must be justified in terms of positive patient outcomes. The time has come to move away from the 'outdated, ritualistic' practices that are 'lacking in fact or research' (Walsh and Ford 1989) and demonstrate insight into what we are doing and why.

Student exercises

• What factors would influence the choice of an expensive treatment option?
• What training would be required to prepare a nurse to apply VAC therapy?
• Consider the aesthetics of having larval therapy.

CHAPTER NINE

Managing infected wounds

The implications of wound infection

A wound infection is defined as one of the complications that adversely affect the wound-healing process (Davis et al. 1992). Wound infection and breakdown of surgical and traumatic wounds still account for a considerable amount of misery, prolonged hospital stay and expense in nursing time, dressings and antibiotics (Westaby and White 1985).

Wound infection is a serious problem and can lead to septicaemia and death. Emmerson et al. (1996) found a prevalence of 10.7% in the Second National Prevalence Survey of Infection in Hospitals, a decrease compared with the 1980 survey when a prevalence of 18.9% was found.

Traditional approaches to identifying infection in wounds involved noting the presence of pus or pus with inflammation (Meers et al. 1980), which is a narrow view considering the range of signs that patients may exhibit. All wounds are inhabited by a multiplicity of bacteria but it is difficult to base a judgement on microbiological assessment alone as to whether a wound is colonized or infected. The patient risk factors mentioned will strongly influence whether or not a wound will become infected and whether or not infection will delay healing (Cutting 1998). Cutting (1998) suggests that diagnosis of infection should be made from a combination of the clinical signs present and laboratory investigations used to identify the offending organism.

Identification of infection in surgically created wounds is fairly straightforward and may present as an abscess with cellulitis and serous, seropurulent, haemopurulent discharge or pus under pressure as the volume increases. Pus consists of a collection of necrotic tissue, bacteria and white cells. Cellulitis occurs as a spreading inflammation of the skin and subcutaneous tissues. Pain, tenderness, erythema, oedema and local heat may be accompanying signs. In severe cases, ulceration, necrosis and pustules may appear. Lymphangitis and enlarged lymph nodes may also be present. A combination of serous discharge and inflammation may be indicative of infection (Leigh 1981), whereas the presence of seropurulent or haemopurulent discharge is the most widely accepted indication of wound infection (Cutting and Harding 1994). Pus is sometimes confused with slough because it can present in various shades similar to slough. There is normally a very distinctive texture to slough that will distinguish it from the more freely flowing liquid or semi-solid pus. The treatment of surgical wound infections is usually simple, involving promotion of drainage of infected material and good wound hygiene or in more severe cases systemic antibiotics (Cutting 1998).

Indicators of wound infection

Infected chronic wounds such as leg ulcers and pressure ulcers are said to constitute an extremely large part of the workload of the primary care team (Gilchrist and Morison 1992). Contamination of any wound with bacteria is inevitable and not necessarily a problem. The body's immune system and phagocytes are designed to deal with contamination. Infection occurs when the contaminating organisms, for a variety of reasons, overwhelm the body defence systems, establish themselves in the wound and multiply.

Reasons why this happens may be one of the following:

- weakened or absent immune response resulting from congenital or systemic disease or immunosuppressant therapy
- systemic disease such as cancer, diabetes or anaemia
- inadequate nutrition.

At the cellular level, infections have four main effects on healing:

1. Fibroblast activity is discouraged, leading to reduced collagen formation plus leukocytes release lysozymes that destroy existing collagen, resulting in a weakened wound.
2. Infection may cause the formation of abscesses in the wound.
3. There is competition between the infecting organisms and the body cells for nutrients and oxygen.
4. The additional demand on the already stretched inflammatory mechanism interferes with normal healing progress.

In summary:

- Infection stops the wound healing.
- The body reacts to the normal presence of bacteria, producing predictable host reactions that assist the practitioner to decide whether or not a wound is infected.

The host reactions are those of inflammation and classically show as heat, pain, swelling and redness, and sometimes pyrexia and pus. These signs are easy to identify in an acute surgical wound in a healthy young person, but less obvious in the case of chronic wounds particularly in elderly people (Gilchrist 1993), those with a compromised immune system caused by illness or taking steroid therapy or those who are neutropenic (Cutting and Harding 1994). In chronic wounds there are often more subtle indicators of infection, such as a sudden increase in exudate levels (this may result from other factors, such as heart failure or uncontrolled venous hypertension – Gilchrist and Morison 1992), that are difficult to cope with.

In the presence of infection, pain may increase or change in nature in and around the wound, but it may also indicate ischaemic changes or vasculitis. Granulation tissue in a healing wound may change in appearance from a healthy bright-red colour to a dusky colour, become more easily damaged and bleed more readily.

Certain infecting organisms can be identified by their distinctive appearance and aroma, e.g. the fluorescent greenish colour seen on dressings from wounds infected with *Pseudomonas aeruginosa*. The characteristic odour of *Pseudomonas aeruginosa* has been described as 'musty'. Wounds infected with staphylococci emit a distinctive putrid smell that is difficult to forget.

All these factors will influence both systemic and local therapy. If infection is confirmed, decisions must be made about whether antibiotics are required, the type of antibiotic and the route of administration. Dressings will be selected according to their level of absorbency, odour-controlling properties, de-sloughing properties, ability to adhere to different parts of the body, bacteria-reducing properties and protective properties to reduce trauma to the wound surface.

Infection in chronic wounds

The diagnosis of infection in chronic wounds such as leg ulcers and pressure ulcers left to heal by secondary intention is more difficult because the signs are more subtle. Infection in chronic wounds often does not exhibit the expected signs of infection, particularly in elderly people and those taking steroid medications, which can lead to confusion and under- or over-treatment.

Cutting and Harding (1994) suggest the following additional criteria to assist in the identification of infection in granulating wounds:

• delayed healing (compared with the normal rate for site/condition)
• discoloration: dull or dark red with patches of necrotic tissue

- friable granulation tissue that bleeds unexpectedly: gelatinous texture gives the wound a raw, red appearance
- unexpected tenderness/pain: caused by swelling and increased tension resulting from tissue fluid
- pocketing at the base of the wound: caused by islands of infection impeding the formation of granulation tissue (Marks et al. 1985)
- bridging of the epithelium: as above, leading to an apparently healed tissue but blue and fragile, which will break down easily
- abnormal smell: anaerobic infections produce a characteristic putrid or acrid smell, e.g. *Pseudomonas aeruginosa*; the presence of necrotic tissue will often cause unpleasant odours
- wound breakdown: this may result from micro-organisms weakening the repaired tissue (Irvin 1981a) or undue stress on the wound
- increased wetness: a sudden increase in exudate may indicate infection, because granulation tissue is relatively dry (Gilchrist 1999). In patients with leg ulcers excessive wetness caused by heart failure must be distinguished from that associated with infection.

There is the constant threat of chronic wounds, and wounds left to heal by secondary intention, becoming infected. At a local level, wound infection stops a wound from healing by (Gilchrist 1999):

- prolonging the inflammatory phase
- depleting the components of the complement cascade
- disrupting normal clotting mechanisms
- interfering with the formation of granulation tissue (Robson et al. 1990).

Systemic effects of wound infection

The effects of bacterial infection vary greatly. At one end of the spectrum there may be delayed healing, temporary disability at the wound site, prolonged hospital stay and temporary loss of productive activity, whereas, at the other extreme, septicaemia and death may be the outcome of a wound infection. The most common cause of death in burns patients was found to be wound infection (Evans 1975). At a cellular level, the mechanism by which bacteria interfere with wound healing is not clear. Systemic symptoms of infection will vary with the age of the patient. In the newborn, other signs such as refusal to feed or jaundice may be the primary indicators of infection. In elderly people a generalized septicaemia or wound breakdown may be the first indications that infection is present (Westaby and White 1985). The type and virulence of the organism, the extent of the infection and the condition of the patient will influence the degree to which infection will spread or be dealt with by the patient's own body defences.

There are several physiological reactions that may occur even if the infection remains localized. Bacterial toxins may cause alterations in cardiac function as a result of increased cardiac output caused by pyrexia. Peripheral vasodilatation may present causing depleted circulating blood volume. Infection may also cause impairment of renal and pulmonary function. Organ dysfunction results from activation of the complement cascade as part of the body's defence mechanism. There is evidence from animal studies that bacteria interfere with collagen synthesis (Niinikoski et al. 1972), and decrease the amount of available oxygen (Bullen et al. 1966) at the wound site, leading to decreased local metabolism and the death of tissue (Irvin 1981a).

Long-term infection depletes the body of nutrients and fluids resulting in catabolism, which leads to rapid weight loss and decreased bacterial resistance, all of which obviously adversely affect wound healing (Westaby and White 1985).

To the patient a wound infection may mean increased pain, frequent dressing changes as a result of high exudate levels, temporary or permanent disability and unpleasant odours, and result in a reluctance to socialize with other people.

The impact of infection on healing tissue

There may be heavy contamination with debris and bacteria following damage to tissue, and bacterial contamination can affect healing in several ways. The inflammatory phase of healing, which lasts for approximately 3–5 days, is a non-specific local response to both tissue damage and bacterial invasion.

The immune system defends the body from bacterial invasion and infection, with all components of the immune system influencing the healing process. The most influential cells in the immune response are the lymphocytes, monocytes and macrophages, with other cells, keratinocytes, endothelial cells and fibroblasts, having a relatively minor part to play. Macrophages are specialized phagocytic cells that produce chemical mediators. During the inflammatory phase they lyse clots and debris and destroy and remove bacteria (Collins et al. 2002). The function of this phase of healing is to cleanse the wound of debris and bacteria, through a series of actions orchestrated by the immune system, and to initiate the production of collagen from fibroblasts found in the wound matrix.

Pathogenic bacteria release an enzyme called collagenase that digests collagen fibres and, in this way, healing is disrupted and the strength of scar tissue impaired. The normal process of the formation of collagen needs an adequate oxygen and nutrient supply; infection, with rapidly dividing aerobic bacteria, will cause competition for oxygen and nutrients and therefore impede healing progress (Gould 1987).

Colonization or infection: how infection is diagnosed

The presence of bacteria on the surface of the wound but not penetrating deeper is known as colonization. All wounds are colonized with bacteria, which does not mean that all wounds will become infected; this is dependent on the host reaction to the bacteria. Skin wounds are colonized by a range of bacteria, including streptococci, staphylococci and *Pseudomonas* sp., and fungi that may cause wound infection.

It is only when bacteria invade into deeper tissues in sufficient numbers to produce symptoms that infection is present. Toxins produced by bacteria can cause local or systemic effects such as septicaemia, which may be fatal.

The four fundamental clinical symptoms of inflammation are: heat, erythema (redness), pain (new or increased) and swelling.

Other signs may include increased exudate, exudate containing pus, local warmth, malaise, fever, high white cell count and loss of function of the injured area. In a sutured surgical wound, the signs are usually minimal and short-lived; in traumatic wounds with extensive damage inflammation is intensified and prolonged by infection. An infected red, hot, oedematous area of skin is called cellulitis and is commonly found in the lower legs in elderly people (Davis et al. 1992).

If clinical infection is suspected by the observation of a number of clinical signs, a wound swab should be taken for culture and sensitivity. Gilchrist (1999) warns that false positives are not uncommon and describes ways in which the reliability of swab reports can be improved, i.e. the careful collection of specimens for anaerobic culture and rapid processing. A wound biopsy is said to be more reliable but is more costly and often impractical. Consultation with the local laboratory service is recommended, particularly about the value of repeated swabbing of chronic wounds which will always be heavily colonized. The effects of localized wound infection can be very serious and lead to non-healing extension of tissue damage and wound dehiscence; at the least, it can cause unacceptable scarring.

Patient assessment

Consideration of any obvious patient risk factors should be the first step with eradication or minimization attempted before local treatment is initiated. The appropriate antibiotics should be prescribed for systemic administration and the course completed. This sounds straightforward but in practice there are many potential complications. There are problems associated with the physical administration of medication to very old and very young people, the cost of treatment, the effects that antibiotics may have on the patient, and whether the most appropriate antibiotics have been prescribed when there is a multiplicity of organisms. Patient compliance with completing the course of antibiotic therapy is a major factor, particularly when patients have been discharged from hospital.

Total eradication of bacteria from a wound is neither desirable nor practical, and there is no evidence that the use of prophylactic antibiotics improves healing rates (Mertz and Eaglstein 1984, Gilchrist and Reed 1989).

Gilchrist (1999) suggests the following as factors that contribute to decreased resistance to infection and which can result in a chronic, non-healing wound:

- the presence of a foreign body in the wound
- the presence of necrotic tissue
- contused tissue
- previous or current irradiation
- presence of a haematoma
- the use of vasoconstricting drugs.

Medical conditions that predispose patients to infection are:

- diabetes
- cancer
- rheumatoid arthritis
- excessive alcohol intake
- malnourishment
- conditions that lead to suppressed or non-functioning of the immune system
- systemic use of steroids or antibiotics
- coexisting distant lesions such as exfoliative dermatitis.

There are several other risk factors associated with clinical practice:

- obesity (Martens et al. 1995): a study of almost 2500 women after a caesarean section
- the length of preoperative stay in hospital: the shorter the stay the less likely is the patient to suffer a wound infection (Cruse and Foord 1980).
- bed occupancy: more than 25 beds in an open ward increased the incidence of infection (Bibby et al. 1986)
- type of surgery (Dealey 2000, based on Cruse and Foord 1980): includes a table to show the types of surgery and respective infection rates (Table 9.1)
- preoperative shaving: a higher rate of wound infection has been found in patients who are shaved preoperatively (Cruse and Foord 1980, Mishriki et al. 1990, Moro et al. 1996 – cited by Dealey 2000). It is suggested that a person be shaved as near to the time of surgery as possible to reduce the risk of infection.

Table 9.1 Classification of surgical wounds

Wound type	Description	Infection rate (%)
Clean	Surgery where there was no infection seen, no break in asepsis and hollow muscular organs not entered. Could include hysterectomy, cholecystectomy or appendicectomy 'in passing' if no evidence of inflammation	1.5
Clean contaminated	Where a hollow muscular organ is entered, but only minimal spillage of contents	7.7
Contaminated	Where a hollow organ was opened with gross spillage of contents, acute inflammation without pus found, a major break in asepsis or traumatic wounds < 4 h old	15.2
Dirty	Traumatic wounds > 4 h old. Surgery where a perforated viscus or pus is found	40

Wound assessment

Comprehensive wound assessment should reveal information about the state of the wound and its clinical appearance. This information will be used to inform appropriate treatment decisions. Questions to the patient may reveal that what the nurse has identified as the main problem is not the patient's main problem. While the nurse concentrates on how to débride the wound, the patient may be more concerned about their soiled clothes from the excess exudate and worries about who will wash them.

Managing infected wounds

The local use of topical antibiotics is not recommended for treating infected wounds (Drugs and Therapeutics Bulletin 1991). They are potentially hazardous and not always absorbed into the wound (Dealey 2000). There are, however, exceptions, such as mupirocin which is recommended for the local treatment of small lesions or skin lesions colonized with methicillin-resistant *Staphylococcus aureus* (MRSA) (Hospital Infection Society 1998), but only for 7–10 days and in line with standard infection control measures (Dealey 2000). There have been reports of mupirocin resistance (Cookson 1998); the author proposes that a more judicious approach to its use be adopted. Another exception is the use of topical metronidazole for malodorous fungating lesions to control the odour of anaerobic bacteria very effectively (Editorial 1990). Silver sulfadiazine, presented as a cream (Flamazine 1%), is very effective against a wide range of bacteria. It has been used for many years to treat minor burns and more recently for treating leg ulcers, and is effective against *Pseudomonas aeruginosa* (Dealey 2000). However, there is some controversy about whether this treatment has any benefit over the use of occlusive dressings (Hutchinson 1992)

Disadvantages of antibacterial agents

Selwyn (1981, cited by Gilchrist 1999) suggests that the use of topical antibacterial agents may lead to:

- local cell and tissue damage
- systemic toxicity
- the development of sensitivity and allergic reactions
- disturbances in the normal skin ecology, leading to superinfection and the possibility of antibiotic resistance
- interactions with other concurrent drug therapies, particularly steroids.

Local policies for antibiotic use should be followed.

Cleansing infected wounds

The aims of wound cleansing are to remove any foreign matter such as gravel or soil, any loose surface debris such as necrotic material and the remnants of the previous dressing (Dealey 2000). However, Thomlinson (1987) demonstrated that the action of cleansing did not reduce the number of bacteria, merely redistributed them. Traditionally, antiseptics such as EUSOL and chlorhexidine have been used to cleanse wounds but Russell et al. (1982) proved that antiseptics would need to be in contact with the wound for 20 minutes before they destroyed bacteria. There are various disadvantages associated with the use of antiseptics for wound cleansing; some general disadvantages are given below. They are rapidly inactivated when they come into contact with body fluids or organic material (Morgan 1993), they can cause irritation and sensitivity, and they are cytotoxic to new cells (Lineaweaver et al. 1985). To summarize, there is little to recommend the use of antiseptics for routine wound cleansing; some have limited use for the initial cleansing of traumatic wounds. Dealey (2000) recommends 0.9% saline as the only completely safe cleansing agent; it is the treatment of choice for cleansing most wounds. Saline is supplied in sachets, plastic tubes and aerosols, which are suitable for irrigating wounds.

Dressing infected wounds

In cases of infected wounds where there is pus, this should be encouraged to drain freely by incising or removing sutures. If necrotic tissue or slough is present, it should be débrided either surgically or autolytically (use of a fluid-donating product or one that maintains a moist environment). The presence of devitalized tissue or any other foreign body in a wound provides an ideal environment for bacteria to flourish (Haury et al. 1980).

The same principles of wound assessment and dressing choice will govern selection for an infected wound as used for a non-infected wound, except that consideration of factors such as high exudate levels or malodour will dominate. Infected wounds are usually wet wounds; control of odour and excess exudate is paramount when dealing with an infected wound.

There is now a wide range of primary and secondary dressings designed for their capacity for absorbency, or for their abilities to attract bacteria from a wound or to deal with odours effectively.

Absorbent dressings

High absorbency profiles can be obtained using one of the adhesive or non-adhesive polyurethane foam products, e.g. Allevyn, CombiDERM, Biatain, Tielle, and Alginate dressings such as Kaltostat, Sorbsan, Tegagen. Cutinova Cavity, Vacutex, Exu-Dry and hydrofibre (Aquacel) products are also highly absorbent and suitable for heavy to moderately exuding wounds. The frequency of dressing change will depend on the volume of exudate and whether the dressing can be retained in place. It is advisable to check an infected wound daily while exudate levels are high and malodour is a problem (Thomas 1990). As with all products the cost-effectiveness of their use must be considered.

Antibacterial dressings

Iodine dressings (Iodoflex, Iodosorb, Inadine) have been shown to reduce the number of bacteria on infected and colonized wounds (Hillstrom 1988, Danielson et al. 1997).

Odour-absorbing dressings

These include Actisorb Silver and Carboflex. The modes of action are sophisticated and slightly different for each, e.g. Carboflex is a primary dressing with a hydrocolloid and alginate wound contact surface, central activated charcoal pad and outer water-resistant outer layer. Actisorb Silver is a primary dressing consisting of an activated charcoal centre impregnated with silver, to which the bacteria are said to be attracted, and trapped within the dressing.

There has been a recent resurgence of interest in the use of silver for its antibacterial properties in wound care as a result of increasing problems associated with antibiotic resistance (White 2001). Silver sulfadiazine has been used to treat burns and grafted areas for many years for its effectiveness against *Pseudomonas aeruginosa* and haemolytic streptococci (Fakhry et al. 1995). Silver nitrate has traditionally been used to treat overgranulation in wounds.

A wide range of silver-containing products is available as hydrocolloid, foam, film, hydrofibre dressings and wound contact layers. White (2001) suggests the following as characteristics of the ideal silver dressing:

• delivers silver in a sustained therapeutic way into the wound
• combined antimicrobial effect and capacity to absorb exudate
• has an odour-control function
• easy and comfortable for the patient
• cost-effective.

The mode of action of silver-containing dressings is primarily down to the continuous release of small amounts of antimicrobial silver into the wound to inhibit the growth of bacteria. The potential value of dressings containing silver is currently attracting a lot of interest and they could have an increasing role in managing antibiotic-resistant wound infection effectively.

Modern wound management products can be used in conjunction with antibiotics but certain products such as Duoderm, Granuflex, Tegaderm and Tegasorb are not recommended for use on clinically infected wounds (Surgical Materials Testing Laboratory Dressing Data Cards: www.smtl.co.uk). The manufacturers do not discount their use, but add the caveat that arrangements for close monitoring of the wound, medical supervision of the patient, adjunctive therapy and daily dressing change should be in place.

There are therapies other than dressing products that will cope with the high exudate and malodour of infected wounds. Reports of the successful use of larval therapy for a wide range of infected wound types from carbuncles to diabetic foot ulcers are presented in the literature (Thomas 1998). The malodour that accompanies infected wounds disappears along with the necrotic tissue as the larvae débride the wound very quickly and effectively. Vacuum-assisted closure (VAC) aids healing of infected wounds in four ways:

1. providing a moist environment to promote cellular activity
2. preventing bacterial contamination from outside the wound
3. evacuating excess wound exudate and bacteria into a canister away from the patient
4. killing anaerobic bacteria in the wound bed.

Collier (1997) reported a reduction in bacterial wound colonization of 1000 times in 4 days with VAC therapy. Again, personal experience of the VAC system has proved that odour decreases and exudate is controlled very effectively by the system.

Honey was the most popular drug as far back as Egyptian times for wound care. The hygroscopic effect of honey when applied to a wound is to starve bacteria of water. Hydrogen peroxide is liberated by an enzyme reaction and produces the antibacterial action. Honey is prone to contamination so it must be sterile when used clinically (Morgan 1997).

Frequently, excess exudate from the infected wound is the most difficult symptom to manage, often the area around the wound becomes painful, macerated and excoriated. Maceration is the softening of tissue that has been moist or wet for a long time (Collins et al. 2002). The skin is white and soggy and more easily damaged. The moisture may be excess exudate from the wound combined with the inability of the dressing to absorb and manage large amounts of exudate. Maceration may also arise from incontinence of urine when it is left in contact with the skin. Excoriation occurs when the skin has been abraded or rubbed away, often in the presence of maceration, as a result of incontinence or inadequate dressings causing wetness around the wound margins (Collins et al. 2002). There are several effective skin barrier preparations now available both for prevention of excoriation in the form of cream and barrier film for prophylaxis and for treatment of maceration and excoriation. The best way, of course, is to anticipate and prevent it happening.

Methicillin-resistant *Staphylococcus aureus*

The discovery, unpredictability and tenacity of MRSA has had a major impact on health care in terms of cost, suffering and the alarm caused by the media. Recent figures show that 100 000 patients acquire infections p.a. while in hospital, costing the NHS approximately £150 million a year. Of these 15% are estimated to be preventable (Denham 2000). The cost of containing a serious outbreak was estimated at between £400 000 and £700 000 in 1998 (Working Party Report 1998).

The origins of staphylococcal resistance to methicillin have been traced back to the first UK and Danish outbreaks in the 1950s, and MRSA is now viewed as the primary cause of potentially life-threatening hospital-acquired infections throughout the world. Infection with *Staphylococcus aureus* has been recognized as a global problem since the 1960s and has been responsible for many serious outbreaks of infection over the last 25 years (DeSaxe et al. 1983, Murray-Leisure et al. 1990, Haley 1991).

The first MRSA infection was identified in a British hospital in 1961 within a year of the introduction of methicillin antibiotics. This was followed in 1963 by the detection of staphylococci in bloodstream infections in Denmark. Both isolates were found to be identical. These findings were running in parallel with the discovery of resistant traits to penicillin, streptomycin, tetracycline and erythromycin. The offending resistant strain of the bacterium has spread throughout hospitals in Belgium, Spain, Portugal, France, Scotland, Germany, Poland, Japan and the USA. The first reports of EMRSA (epidemic MRSA) were from inner-London hospitals in 1981; since then, EMRSA has continued to develop until now EMRSA15 and EMRSA16 are common.

Unfortunately, newer, stronger, rapidly spreading strains are reaching epidemic levels. The rates are lowest in those countries that have strict infection control policies and highest in those with liberal policies; however, the general trend is towards more resistance. The number of patients infected or colonized with MRSA continues to rise in the UK. Casewell (1995) reported that up to 60% of *Staphylococcus aureus* infections were methicillin resistant. Control and management are very costly as a result of the high numbers of patients involved, the high cost of vancomycin for treatment and prophylaxis (Casewell 1995), and the emerging resistance to newer antibiotics. Different strains cause different problems for patients: EMRSA3 is frequently isolated from pressure ulcers, EMRSA16 is commonly associated with pulmonary infections and EMRSA15 appears to favour people in elderly care units (Duckworth and Heathcock 1995). The range of antibiotics to which the newer strains are sensitive is narrow and decreasing fast.

Staphylococcus aureus

Bacteria are single-celled organisms that are found everywhere; they usually perform useful roles within the body as normal flora (organisms that normally live in or on the human body) and control the potential overgrowth of other organisms. However, bacteria also constitute the largest group of pathogens (micro-organisms that cause disease). Bacteria are grouped according to their shape: coccus (spheroidal or round), bacillus (rod-shaped) and curved rod shaped. Cocci are usually arranged in patterns such as pairs, chains, bunches of grapes or clusters. All bacteria are capable of independent functions regarding reproduction and the maintenance of life. Most species of bacteria are non-pathogenic compared with the numbers found free living. Most of those found in hospital are described as opportunistic, i.e. they are virulent enough to attack the tissues of frail, debilitated people and cause clinical disease. Hospitals, housing large numbers of vulnerable individuals, therefore have become ideal environments in which bacteria flourish.

The cocci cause diseases such as gonorrhoea, meningitis, pneumonia and rheumatic fever. Healthy people may be the unsuspecting carriers of potentially pathogenic bacteria such as *Staphylococcus aureus* in their axillae, nose, groin, toe webs and perineum. *Staphylococcus aureus* exists in the nasal mucosa of approximately 30% of the adult population, in the faeces of about 20% and on the skin of approximately 5–10%, and even higher percentages in hospital workers (Gould 1987). Carriers may be responsible for the infection of vulnerable individuals or people who have undergone surgical or other invasive procedures if the normal protective barriers of the skin are breached and, therefore, represent a potential threat to others. The intact skin not only provides a physical barrier against infection, but also contains immunological cells, lymphoid and Langerhans' cells, and cells that produce a number of immunity-modulating substances as demonstrated in the inflammatory response to tissue damage. The dry, impermeable surface of the stratum corneum constitutes the major physical barrier because it is inhospitable to most pathogenic organisms, but when it is over-hydrated or disrupted it can predispose to bacterial invasion. Pathogenic organisms can reach the skin by either external or internal routes although the external route is more common for skin infections.

Staphylococcus aureus is a Gram-positive bacterium that is a normal human commensal present on the skin surface. Bacteria are shed from the skin of carriers and become trapped in bedclothes and clothes, and on medical equipment. *Staphylococcus aureus* is transmitted mainly via the hands and fingers (Bradley 1985), hence the need for adequate hand washing. As a result of its ability to synthesize a range of protective enzymes, the bacterium is capable of rapid spread; this function prevents the bacterium being attacked and destroyed by the host white blood cells, making it a highly successful and adaptable pathogen.

Most bacterial infections of the skin are caused by *Staphylococcus aureus* or group A β-haemolytic streptococci (*Streptococcus pyogenes*), which gain entry via traumatized skin or hair follicles producing chemotactic factors that attract neutrophils. This can result in pus formation, and the release of enzymes that contribute to the inflammatory response. The cocci cause diseases such as gonorrhoea, meningitis, pneumonia and rheumatic fever, wound infections and less serious conditions such as infected cuts and boils.

Risk factors for MRSA

The problem of MRSA in nursing homes has been recognized in the USA for several years but little has been published in the UK (Goodall and Tomkins 1994). MRSA is primarily a problem of hospital cross-infection where staff or fellow patients, as carriers, present a threat to contacts. The risk of acquiring MRSA is linked to length of stay and frequency of re-admission to hospital, the presence of pressure ulcers, physiotherapy, catheters, the use of intravascular devices and surgical procedures (Crowcroft et al. 1996). Very young people, those aged between 60 and 71 years and immunocompromised people have been found to be most at risk of death from MRSA sepsis (Locksley 1982, Dunk-Richards 1985). However, Meers and Leong (1990), when discussing control measures, state that MRSA is no more pathogenic than its methicillin-sensitive counterpart. Layton et al. (1995) found that 41% of hospitalized patients have community-acquired infections. The risk factors associated with community acquisition of MRSA were recent hospitalization, previous antibiotic therapy, nursing home residence, increased numbers of day cases and intravenous drug use. Casewell (1995) believes that we have created a 'new reservoir' of infected and colonized patients because of a high incidence of pressure ulcers and leg ulcers in residents. The decrease in the number of hospital beds means that colonized and infected patients are rapidly transferred back to nursing and residential homes after treatment.

The evidence that MRSA poses a significant problem in nursing and residential homes is patchy and incomplete, but the risk of colonized patients being transferred between hospital and community should not be underestimated (Duckworth and Heathcock 1995). Precautions should be taken regarding the MRSA status of patients transferring between hospital and community, until screening proves negative. Duckworth and Heathcock (1995) believe that MRSA in nursing and residential homes usually takes the form of colonization rather than infection and poses little or no threat to other residents. The Department of Health (DoH) published an information booklet in 1996 clarifying MRSA and its implications for nursing and residential home residents. The need for information was prompted by concern about patients with MRSA being discriminated against and being refused admission to nursing and residential homes. The booklet provides clear guidance about hygiene precautions and the housing of MRSA-positive residents, e.g. sharing a room with a person who has no open sores, wounds, drips or catheters, and appropriate dressings for wounds.

The emphasis is on normality for the resident as far as possible and good basic hygiene to prevent infections:

- Good hand hygiene practice by staff and residents is the single most important infection control measure.
- Disposable gloves and aprons should be worn when attending to dressings, performing aseptic techniques or dealing with blood and body fluids.
- Cuts, sores or wounds in staff and residents should be covered with impermeable dressings.
- Blood and body fluid spills should be dealt with immediately according to locally agreed policy.

- Sharps should be disposed of into proper sharps containers.
- Equipment such as commodes should be cleaned thoroughly with detergent and hot water after use.
- Clothes and bedding should be machine washed, in accordance with the local policy.
- Cutlery, crockery and clinical waste should be dealt with in the normal way (DoH 1996).

Other recommendations include informing the hospital before admission or outpatient treatment at the hospital that the resident has MRSA and obtaining advice from the local microbiologist or infection control nurse.

The psychological effects of MRSA and its treatment should not be underestimated. In hospital, patients are often isolated or at least treated differently to non-infected patients. They may feel ostracized or different in some way to other patients. Isolation in the community is not recommended because it may interfere with the person's rehabilitation. However, in a recent small-scale study individual response to isolation was found to be variable; some patients experienced emotional disturbance but others expressed a preference for being hospitalized in a single room. Of those experiencing negative emotional effects of isolation, improved communication and facilities were identified as key factors (Ward 2000). Isolating patients may be seen as the demands of the organization being more important than those of the patient (Olsen 1992). Clinicians should be well informed about the necessary precautions and able to educate the patient and carers about transmission and hygiene measures during admission and before discharge from hospital. Reassurance that transmission to family members or other residents is a rare occurrence must be given.

Recognition of control of MRSA as a major problem in hospitals led to guidelines being published in 1998 (Working Party Report 1998), followed by the UK Antimicrobial Resistance Strategy and Action Plan (DoH 2000). The impetus to reconvening the Working Party, which originally met in 1995, was the increased prevalence and changes in epidemiology of MRSA and limited resources to control it. The key to control was thought to be assessment of the degree of risk to patients and their contacts and a more flexible approach dictated by local circumstances.

The Working Party Report (1998) guidelines emphasize good basic practices for controlling MRSA.

Management

- surveillance of important organisms
- audit programme that monitors compliance with policies
- adequate staffing levels and skill mix.

Clinical

- clean ward environment
- effective hand hygiene, antiseptic technique and isolation policy
- appropriate use of protective clothing
- compliance with clinical waste, laundry and antibiotics policies
- no patient overcrowding with minimal inter-ward movement.

Clinical pathways for MRSA patients encompassing isolation procedures, ward closure, cleaning and disinfection should be in place. However, recognizing that there are variations between different localities, it was recommended that decisions should be based on local circumstances, clinical experience, available resources, whether the situation is epidemic or endemic, and the vulnerability of other patients. High-risk areas were identified as intensive care, neonatal units, orthopaedics and trauma units, whereas low-risk areas were medical and elderly care and mental health facilities. Recommendations for a screening protocol, the treatment of carriers and those with infected/colonized skin lesions are also included.

The key elements to controlling antimicrobial resistance, suggested by the Department of Health (2000), are surveillance to inform action, prudent antimicrobial use and infection control to reduce the spread of infection. These elements should be supported by tailored information, education, communication, research, the necessary infrastructure, organizational support and legislation, where necessary.

Wilson (1995) concluded that the best way to control the spread of MRSA was to treat the infection or eradicate colonization as quickly as possible. Screening and treatment practices vary between organizations; some screen and isolate all MRSA patients whereas others may do so only in specific circumstances. Only those patients found to be at risk for MRSA should be screened, and where there is likely to be a recognized benefit to the patient or an identifiable risk to other patients (Forrest 2000). This will lead to better patient care generally, but, in particular, will cause less inconvenience to patients and staff, and reduce costs.

Basic principles of care and common sense should be the foundation for all nursing practice. Wound management will vary according to the site of damage, whether it is colonized or infected, and the sensitivity pattern of the MRSA. Comprehensive, holistic assessment of the patient is essential to identify the factors that may influence the risk of infection and the outcome of management. Dressings should be applied away from other at-risk patients after hand washing, and using gloves, gowns and sterile dressings. Swabbing the wound for MRSA is unnecessary unless the wound is deteriorating or new wounds are appearing in a patient at risk. General microbiological investigations are recommended in these situations, with information to the laboratory that the patient has or has had MRSA infection, if appropriate.

MRSA colonization does not usually require an aggressive approach; however, a systemic MRSA infection may result in potentially fatal complications such as endocarditis, osteomyelitis or pneumonia in a vulnerable patient. The presence of bacteria in a wound does not necessarily prevent healing (Gilchrist and Reed 1989), but the presence of infection in a wound can impede it (Gilchrist and Morison 1992), although how this happens is unclear. Suspicion of clinical infection in a wound may be based on the following signs: heat, redness, swelling, increased pain, increased exudate, pus, changes in the appearance of granulation tissue and odour. Clinical infection in chronic wounds in elderly people, such as leg ulcers and pressure ulcers, may not be immediately obvious as a result of a deficient immune response to infection. Laboratory results can identify the micro-organism present in the wound, whether it is colonized or infected, and support the diagnosis with the presence of pus on microscopy. However, microbiological samples may not provide any growth on culture although this does not rule out the presence of clinical infection. Local policies will dictate the circumstances under which wound swabs should be taken.

As with any wound suspected of being infected or colonized, systematic assessment and knowledge of wound management principles are prerequisites for a successful outcome. If a wound is colonized, care must be taken to provide the optimum conditions for healing, which will include general patient support, the provision of a moist healing environment and prevention of the spread of bacteria. This can be achieved by occluding the wound with an occlusive dressing such as a hydrocolloid (Duckworth and Heathcock 1995), which, in theory, can be left in place for up to 7 days, in the absence of clinical infection.

Clinically infected wounds pose two main problems: the presence of necrotic tissue blocking the effectiveness of a topical antimicrobial and excess exudate. Necrotic tissue or slough in a wound either should be removed by sharp débridement if appropriate or can be dealt with using a hydrogel covered by a semi-permeable film dressing or a hydrocolloid dressing to rehydrate the devitalized tissue. Exudate can be dealt with using one of the many absorbent wound management products now available. These include foams, alginates, paste cavity fillers or capillary action dressings. There is also a place for VAC therapy which draws excess exudate via a closed system into a sealed canister, thereby reducing odour and risk of cross-infection. The size, location and severity of the wound will guide product or therapy suitability. Waterproof adhesive dressings will allow for body disinfection and contain bacteria. In the presence of clinical infection and often large volumes of exudate, it is usually prudent, and often necessary, to change dressings daily; the manufacturer's dressing guidelines should be followed.

The debate surrounding the use of topically applied antibacterials continues. Selwyn (1981) believes that topical antimicrobials should not be used because they may:

- cause cell death and tissue damage
- lead to systemic toxicity
- lead to contact sensitivity and allergic reactions
- lead to superinfection and antibiotic resistance
- interact with other therapy such as steroids.

In spite of the above, wounds with MRSA are often treated with topical antimicrobials and/or topical antiseptics. The most commonly used are mupirocin, povidone–iodine, chlorhexidine and silver sulfadiazine. Practice varies between organizations and areas, and there is little agreement about what constitutes the best or most effective treatment. Mupirocin is the antimicrobial agent of choice in most centres and is usually applied twice daily for between 7 and 14 days to minimize the risk of resistance developing (Casewell 1995). Topical silver sulfadiazine and the newer silver-containing dressings are becoming more popular in the management of MRSA-infected wounds. There are claims for the effectiveness of both chlorhexidine and povidone–iodine, used to soak and cleanse wounds, in controlling MRSA (Beedle 1993, Lacey and Catto 1993). There is consensus about limiting the duration of treatment with any antimicrobial or antiseptic preparation to minimize resistance.

Staphylococcus aureus is considered a marker of infection control practices and hospital-acquired infection rates, and MRSA a marker of the prevalence of MRSA infection within that hospital. Measures have been established to tackle the problem of MRSA through data collection, observation of trends and laboratory audit of activity surrounding MRSA, which will be expressed as a proportion of all hospital activity and regular central reporting (DoH 2000). The aim is to determine why there are variances in rates of MRSA and to learn from good practice.

At the practical level, there is still a lot of uncertainty about how best to manage MRSA within a constantly changing picture caused by the emergence of new strains and new antibiotic resistance. It is a complex problem and one that is becoming more difficult and more expensive to contain. With regard to wound management and MRSA, basic principles of wound care and commonsense approaches to achieving consistently high standards of hygiene (hand washing) are vital, combined with an awareness of current debates on this dynamic problem.

In any setting, health-care professionals have a major responsibility for identifying those factors that influence the risk of infection and taking action to safeguard the patient from the effects of infection. This can be done at three levels: the individual patient, organization wide and community wide. At the patient level, steps must be taken to tailor care to specific needs to safeguard the patient, e.g. identify risk factors for infection and act appropriately. At an organizational level, clinicians must adhere to infection control policies and procedures, e.g. good hand-washing technique and observation of isolation measures. At the general community level, there must be support for health-promotion strategies to detect, report and eradicate disease.

Conclusion

The management of patients with infected wounds presents the nurse and patient with many challenges. Patients with infected wounds are likely to be anxious about the progress of their treatment, the outcome, scarring and how they will cope when discharged from hospital. Nurses have the challenges of dealing with the psychological effects on the patient as well as whether they have the specialist practical knowledge and skills to be able to manage the wound appropriately. The clinical treatment of infected wounds is complicated and requires input from many members of the multidisciplinary team, from dietitians, nurses, surgeons and microbiologists to product experts.

Student exercises

- List the main risk factors for increased susceptibility to wound infection.
- What basic precautions should be taken to prevent the spread of bacterial contamination?

CHAPTER TEN

Classification and treatment of different wound types: chronic wounds

This chapter provides a brief overview of chronic wounds treated regularly by the multidisciplinary health-care team. The aetiology, presentation and management options of each are discussed.

Pressure ulcers

The epidemiology of pressure ulcers is described in Chapter 12. The costs, implications, aetiology and clinical management of patients with pressure ulcers are discussed below.

Costs and implications of pressure ulcers

Demographic changes in the population are leading to an explosion in the number of elderly people, with increasing costs associated with age-related conditions. The costs of personnel, consumables, new technologies and therapies, rising public expectations and litigation result in ever greater demands on public expenditure in relation to pressure ulcer development. Although the economic burden of pressure ulcers is largely unknown, it remains difficult to calculate the indirect costs to society as a whole. Direct costs are easier to measure because they relate directly to health service costs; those that fall outside this arena are incalculable.

Various unsubstantiated estimates (McSweeney 1994) of the cost of pressure ulcers have been proposed, from £60 million (Department of Health or DoH 1991) to £300 million (Waterlow 1988). Hibbs (1988) decided to quantify the cost of a pressure ulcer by following up a patient with a necrotic sacral ulcer for 1 year. The result was a figure of £25 000, most of which arose from nursing costs: 26% from management of the pressure ulcer; 17.5% for bed hire; and only 6% on wound care products (Franks 2001). Extended length of hospitalization is estimated to be between 9 and 140 days (Clinical Standards Advisory Group or CSAG

1993), causing lost opportunity to treat other patients but not necessarily higher overall costs. One patient vacating a hospital bed could allow several high-cost patients to pass through using the same bed. Another study calculated that 12% of community nurse visits were to patients for pressure ulcer care, with one-third being daily visits to patients with severe pressure damage (McSweeney 1994).

In 1993 Touche Ross, a firm of accountants, estimated the cost of pressure ulcer treatment alone as between £644 000 and £1 153 000 p.a. and the cost of prevention as £2 710 000 p.a. in an average 600-bed hospital (Touche-Ross Report 1994). All this means is that we are currently unclear about how much money is spent on pressure ulcer prevention and treatment.

Aetiology of pressure ulcers

The working definition of a pressure ulcer is an area of localized damage to the skin and underlying tissues caused by pressure, shear, friction and/or a combination of these (European Pressure Ulcer Advisory Panel or EPUAP 1999). Simply put, pressure ulcers are the clinical manifestation of localized tissue death caused by lack of blood flow in areas subjected to pressure (Sciarra 2003). Pressure ulcers are most commonly found where pressure compresses tissue over a bony prominence in the body – the tissues are pinched between a hard undersurface and the deep bone. There are wide variations in the ability of different tissues to withstand pressure and maintain vascular flow at different pressure intensities. Tissue tolerance is described as the ability of both the skin and its supporting structures to endure the effects of pressure without adverse side sequelae (Braden and Bergstrom 1987). Skin has a comparatively high tolerance to pressure whereas muscle and fat have a low tolerance. Tissue compression impedes blood flow, resulting in ischaemia with reduced or absent delivery of nutrients and oxygen to the cells, which will eventually die producing an area of tissue damage known as a pressure ulcer.

Death of the deeper tissues is difficult to detect until the damage is serious because necrosis occurs at bone level and may take days from the initial insult to reveal itself. In a healthy individual, capillaries are said to fill at 32 mmHg where capillaries connect to arterioles, so external pressure of more than 32 mmHg at this point will cause problems by obstructing blood flow into the capillaries. In the elderly, frail patient, the external capillary closing pressures may be much lower and so cause tissue damage at lower pressures. The converse of this is that the fit body builder will be able to withstand much greater pressures before damage occurs. More research is needed to elicit exact values of capillary closing pressure in the vulnerable person.

In the tissues subjected to pressure for a long enough period, the capillaries will collapse and thrombose, metabolic waste products will accumulate and surrounding cells will start to die deep at bone level. Eventually the external signs will be oedema caused by leakage from the capillaries, and redness and localized heat resulting from blood being forced into the surrounding tissues. The patient may not feel pain until the structures containing nerve endings are affected.

Under normal circumstances, the healthy individual, when subjected to high pressures, will move spontaneously before tissue damage occurs, but in the elderly, infirm, frail person the ability to reposition may be impaired. Low pressure exerted for long periods is more damaging than short bursts of high pressure, when the tissues and vasculature have time to recover. Therefore, elderly, infirm, frail, immobile patients are more likely to succumb to pressure damage because they are less able to move themselves.

The other significant factors that influence the development of pressure damage are shearing forces and friction, often combined with moisture from incontinence, exudate or perspiration. Shearing forces are mechanical forces created either by the body being repositioned or as the patient slides down the bed from a sitting position. Gravity is a key factor because it pulls the body down the bed while the skin resists the movement and stays in contact with the sheets. The underlying tissues and blood vessels are distorted, stretched and crushed, while the external picture is one of puckering of the skin.

The addition of shearing forces to pressure intensifies the effect and damage to the tissues, and reduces the time necessary for damage to happen. Pressure ulcers resulting from pressure and shear are characteristically deep and triangular or teardrop shaped, whereas those principally caused by pressure are usually deep and more circular in shape.

Friction, another mechanical force, has also been implicated as a contributory cause of tissue damage and happens as one surface moves across another, e.g. as the patient rubs a heel on the bedclothes, or, knowingly or unknowingly, when patients are dragged, rather than lifted, across the bed with a low-friction lifting aid.

The risk of frictional damage is higher in those with uncontrollable spasm who wear prostheses or have difficulty clearing the bed surface when they attempt to move themselves. The outcome will be an abrasion or blister over the bony prominence increasing the potential for more serious tissue damage. Moisture will waterlog or macerate the skin and deeper tissues to the point where connective tissue becomes softer and more fragile. The epidermis is more fragile when wet, so damage can occur from contact with the sheet, worsening the effects of frictional forces; moist skin is five times more likely to develop damage than dry skin (Sciarra 2003).

Summary of the causes of pressure ulcers

Pressure ulcers are caused by: pressure, shearing forces and friction, usually combined with moisture – it is usually a combination of two or more of these factors that predispose the patient to tissue breakdown.

Location of pressure ulcers

Pressure ulcers typically occur over bony or cartilaginous prominences. Common locations are: sacrum, ischial tuberosity, coccyx, greater trochanters, heels, elbows, occiput, malleoli, ears.

Two-thirds of pressure ulcers occur in the pelvic girdle as a result of more body weight dependence and bony prominences.

Risk factors for pressure ulcer development

Risk is a word frequently used in relation to pressure ulcer prevention and the likelihood of tissue damage. Ultimately, risk should direct both preventive efforts and treatment plans. Nurses must familiarize themselves with the data that are available relating external and internal risk factors with tissue damage, to enable correction of correctable deficiencies or situations and to ensure that the patient receives the best quality care. According to current research data certain populations appear to be consistently identified as high risk for pressure damage. There is evidence that pressure ulcers are more likely to occur in elderly than in younger patients. However, certain groups such as post-surgery patients, spinal-injured patients and those with darkly pigmented skin have been found to be more vulnerable and to sustain more severe tissue damage (Papantonio et al. 1994, Fuhrer et al. 1993). Gender, however, does not appear to influence the development of pressure ulcers (Van Rijswijk 2001).

Known risk factors for pressure ulcer development include the following:

- Mobility problems: immobility may be the most significant risk factor (David et al. 1983, Nyquist and Hawthorn 1987) and may result from physical or psychological causes. The ability to move spontaneously in response to pressure discomfort may be lost as a result of paralysis, severe illness, mental health problems or sedative and hypnotic medication.
- Poor general health: pre-existing diseases of the cardiovascular system, metabolic disorders and general debility strongly influence the development of tissue damage.
- Acute illness: possibly caused by pain, low blood pressure, heart failure, the use of sedatives, vasomotor failure, shock and others (Bliss 1990).

Patients who are acutely ill move less frequently, and are more likely to be incontinent and have cardiovascular irregularities such as low blood pressure.

- Advancing age: changes to the skin, vascularity and subcutaneous tissue structure and quality with age reduce the ability of the patient to withstand excessive pressure, shearing and frictional forces. Reduction in the efficiency of the immune system also produces a less effective inflammatory response and resistance to infection in the patient.
- Hip and lower limb fracture: Versluysen (1986) found a pressure ulcer prevalence of 66% in a group of 100 patients aged over 60 years.
- Hospitalized patients with paralysis: changes to the normal routine of the paralysed patient can be a major risk factor. Admission to hospital, surgery, unfamiliar support surfaces and erratic dietary intake can be problematic to paralysed patients.
- Poor nutritional status: pre-existing anaemia, malnourishment and low protein levels are associated with pressure ulcer development.
- Presence of incontinence: maceration and frequent cleansing with alkaline soap weakens the protective barrier of the skin, making it more vulnerable to breakdown. Faecal incontinence is often associated with general patient deterioration.
- Diabetes mellitus: the coexistence of peripheral neuropathy and microvascular disease increases the risk of damage.
- Decreased mental status: may lead to poor nutritional intake; sedative and hypnotic medication, and mental state may reduce mobility level.
- Previous history of pressure ulcers: scar tissue is never as strong as the original tissue so, although there may be evidence of good healing, the area will be susceptible to breakdown.
- Peripheral vascular disease, respiratory disease, cancer, i.e. multiple medical conditions: any condition that impedes the delivery of oxygen and nutrients to the cells or interferes with normal cell metabolism will cause cell malnutrition or ischaemia, thus increasing the risk of pressure damage.
- The patient's length of stay in hospital: this may be associated with deteriorating general health, complications resulting from surgery or acute-on-chronic illness. As the patient's stay is extended, so the risk of pressure damage increases possibly caused by poor nutritional intake, prolonged bed-rest or sitting in a chair, combined with losing the will to live and depression.

This list is not exhaustive; in a review of the literature, however, five key themes were identified: mobility, nutrition, perfusion, age and skin condition (Nixon and McGough 2001). Rintala (1995) found associations between pressure ulcers and life satisfaction, quality of life, level of self-esteem and social support in spinal cord-injured patients. Other important considerations include the environment of care, staffing levels and the experience of staff caring for the patients.

Prevention of pressure ulcers

Prevention should be the key word. Most pressure ulcers are preventable, even as the elderly population increases, with the increased knowledge and equipment available. Before the advent of assessment tools for pressure ulcer risk, clinical judgement was used to identify patients at risk of pressure damage; although unscientific, it relied on past experience of the nurse (and doctor), ongoing observation and repositioning schedules. As risk assessment became more sophisticated tools were developed to enhance, not replace, clinical judgement to identify those patients likely to suffer pressure damage.

The general common denominators integrated into risk assessment tools are immobility, inactivity, incontinence, malnutrition and impaired mental status or sensation; there are variations according to the tool chosen. The most commonly used risk calculators today are the Waterlow Risk Assessment Scale in the UK (Waterlow 1985) and the Braden Score in the USA (Bergstrom et al. 1987).

The Waterlow Risk Assessment Scale comprises a number of variables against which the patient is scored, and ends with a calculated risk level: 10+ at risk, 15+ high risk and 20+ very high risk. The score should then be considered when choosing a support surface, e.g. the very-high-risk patient, with or without pressure ulcers, would probably warrant an alternating pressure mattress replacement such as a Nimbus III. The risk assessment scale will not predict who will develop a pressure ulcer; it will identify only patients who are likely, based on the combination of existing risk factors, to be at risk. The risk level will change during admission as patients' general condition improves, as they undergo surgery or invasive investigations, or as they deteriorate.

All patients entering health care, hospital or community should be assessed as early as feasible after first contact, and within 6 hours of admission to hospital (NICE 2001). Urgency is crucial to providing the most appropriate support surface and preventive interventions as early as possible after admission. Re-assessment should be carried out as the patient's condition changes, on transfer between different environments and postoperatively. A holistic approach to prevention is required, taking into account existing and intervening risk factors on a regular basis using formal and informal assessment procedures. Accurate, up-to-date documentation of findings is essential to good communication and consistent care. Risk assessment should be conducted only by individuals who have undergone appropriate training to recognize risk factors and know how to initiate and maintain correct and suitable preventive measures (NICE 2001).

Observation of the skin

An individual who has received training on what to look for and is able to initiate correct preventive measures should carry out skin inspection. The primary nurse should be informed immediately of any changes identified. The most vulnerable areas for each person should be inspected (as listed previously), plus the skin under antiembolism stockings, prostheses in contact with equipment, bandages and plasters. Where possible, patients should be taught how to inspect their skin and encouraged to do so; mirrors may be used by patients using wheelchairs.

What to look for

- Routine skin inspection may reveal dryness, cracking, maceration, fragility, heat, induration, pallor or erythema (redness) which may indicate early ischaemia. Documentation of the initial skin inspection is useful as a baseline description to compare with subsequent changes; later, it will indicate whether preventive measures have been effective in preventing tissue damage. The skin over the bony prominences will obviously be the priority but other areas such as the ears, occiput or skinfolds should also be inspected. Patients with darkly pigmented skin are difficult to assess for changes to the skin colour because these are not visible. Heat, swelling and induration are more reliable indicators of pressure damage in darkly pigmented skin.
- It is vital that the first signs of tissue damage are recognized and acted upon. Early signs in light-skinned people are fixed red marks that do not blanch (go white) after 30 minutes or on the gentle application of finger pressure to the area (non-blanching erythema). Non-blanching erythema is an indication that the microcirculation is damaged and the result will be ischaemia of the surrounding tissues. In patients with dark skin, discomfort, swelling and raised local skin temperature will indicate that damage has occurred.
- The aim of identifying skin changes caused by pressure is to limit the potential for damage by regular re-positioning, good skin care and general patient support such as adequate nutritional intake. The frequency of re-positioning will be dictated by the visible signs of blanching erythema and non-blanching erythema to prevent the damage worsening.
- Vulnerable patients or those with pressure damage should be nursed in bed on an alternating pressure replacement mattress; however, there is

often pressure on nurses to 'mobilize' patients. This should not mean that they are left sitting in a chair for many hours. The recommended time limit for sitting is 2 hours (NICE 2001). Old-fashioned massage and creams are not recommended and may, in fact, increase the risk of damage. Incontinence must be managed by re-training, assisting to the toilet or urinary catheterization, if appropriate.

• Other sources of moisture such as wound exudate and perspiration must be controlled. Skin cleansing with a gently moisturizing, non-soap cleanser is now recommended. Moisturizers and emollients should be used regularly to protect and maintain the skin in good condition. Correct positioning and patient handling are essential to the preservation of healthy skin. Education and training should be provided regularly to all carers on positioning patients and using hoists and other patient-handling devices.

Classifying pressure damage

Pressure ulcers may be divided into two main groups: the first, most serious, type occurs because of prolonged exposure to pressure, experienced internally between the soft tissues and bony prominences, which results in deep damage caused by ischaemia and necrosis (surgical type pressure ulcer). The second, less serious, type occurs in acutely ill patients during short periods of high pressure resulting in superficial skin and tissue damage (medical type).

Several classification systems have been developed that describe the extent of tissue damage to aid communication through documentation. The EPUAP (1999) classification has been widely adopted for its relative simplicity and ease of use:

• Grade 1: non-blanchable erythema of intact skin. Discoloration of the skin, warmth, oedema, induration or hardness may also be used as indicators particularly on individuals with darker skin.
• Grade 2: partial-thickness skin loss involving epidermis, dermis or both. The ulcer is superficial and presents clinically as an abrasion or blister.
• Grade 3: full-thickness skin loss involving damage to, or necrosis of, subcutaneous tissue which may extend down to, but not through, underlying fascia.
• Grade 4: extensive destruction, tissue necrosis or damage to muscle, bone or supporting structures with or without full-thickness skin loss.

It will be noted that the skin is not broken in a grade 1 pressure ulcer. The patient may complain of discomfort at this stage, whereas, as the damage progresses to grade 2, the patient will also start to feel a stinging, painful sensation as the nerve endings are exposed to dryness and cooler temperatures. At the other extreme, the patient with a grade 4 pressure ulcer will often not complain of pain because the nerve endings have been destroyed. The risk of infection is present as soon as the integrity of the skin is breached, from grade 2 to the point where septicaemia becomes a major risk, sometimes resulting in death.

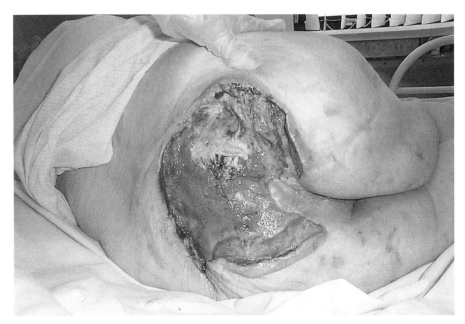

Figure 10.1 Sacral pressure ulceration (see Plate 13).

Management of patients with pressure ulcers

The mainstay of pressure ulcer management is to remove or alleviate the underlying cause by providing the correct support surface, preventing further damage, controlling pain and optimizing the patient's general condition. Every patient should have a personalized written prevention plan to aid communication and recovery. The plan will include frequency of re-positioning, time spent sitting, the type of mattress/seat cushion used and when provided, nutritional assessment/supplementation and evaluation of all related interventions. Patients and their relatives/carers should be given the opportunity to participate in decisions about their care. They should be provided with written and oral information about how to prevent pressure damage and about the special equipment used to prevent and treat pressure ulcers.

Ulcers of the lower leg

The epidemiology of leg ulceration is described in Chapter 12. The aetiology and management of patients with different types of leg ulcers are discussed here.

Leg ulcers are chronic wounds arising from predisposing conditions that impair the ability of the tissue to maintain its integrity or heal damage (Davis et al. 1992). Examples in the lower limb include:

- impaired venous drainage, e.g. venous hypertension
- impaired arterial supply, e.g. peripheral vascular disease
- metabolic abnormalities, e.g. diabetes mellitus.

The outcome will be an established area of epithelial discontinuity (Davis et al. 1992) or ulceration, which may be venous, arterial, neuropathic or associated with other disease processes.

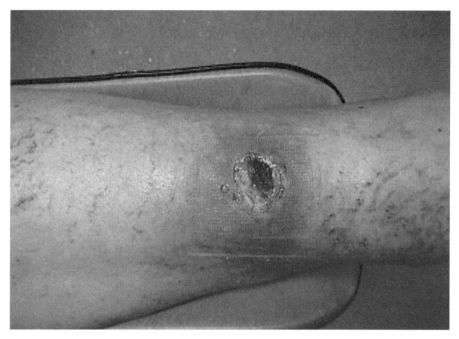

Figure 10.2 Venous leg ulcer (see Plate 14).

Ulceration arising from chronic venous disease accounts for over 70% of leg ulcers and affects 1–2% of the UK population (Laing 1992). The highest prevalence of venous leg ulceration is in very elderly people (Cornwall et al. 1986). The cost to treat patients suffering from venous leg ulceration is estimated to be in the region of £400 million a year (Bosanquet 1992). Treatment is characteristically long term and the rate of recurrence is high.

Aetiology

Damage to the venous valves in the legs may result from deep vein thrombosis or sustained venous hypertension as a result of pregnancy or obesity. The venous return between the superficial system and the deep veins is impeded when the valves cease to function efficiently. Backflow of blood occurs in the superficial system, leading to varicose veins and eventually lipodermatosclerosis (woody induration or fibrosis of the skin and tissues), venous stasis and oedema. Other mechanisms that aid venous return are the calf muscle pump and negative pressure generated in the abdomen and thorax during respiration. Calf muscles aid venous return as they contract and squeeze the veins in the leg, propelling blood back to the heart; as they relax the veins re-fill with blood and the process is repeated. If the calf muscle pump is inactive as a result of paralysis the blood flow is inhibited.

The development of varicose veins, common in nurses and others spending long periods standing in warm environments, should be a warning sign to a small number of individuals of the possibility of tissue breakdown. Several predisposing factors have been identified:

- family history
- certain occupations where people must stand for long periods, e.g. shop assistants
- gender; more common in women than in men with increasing age
- pregnancy
- low-fibre diet
- obesity (Morison and Moffatt 1997)
- reduced mobility in the lower limb.

The signs of venous insufficiency include an ulcer with pitting oedema, brown staining in the gaiter area, ankle flare (dilatation of the tiny superficial veins on the medial aspect of the ankle) and atrophy of the skin; eczema is also commonly found. Patients may complain of a feeling of heaviness, swelling, itchiness, pain and tenderness in the legs. The ulcer will be characteristically located near the medial or lateral malleolus, but may occur anywhere between the ankle and the mid-calf. The venous ulcer is usually shallow and irregularly shaped, and often filled with beefy-looking granulation tissue, but it can be filled with necrotic or sloughy tissue or covered by a yellow film of fibrin. Hyperpigmentation resulting from the breakdown of leaked red blood cells in the tissues may be evident. Atrophie blanche may appear as sometimes painful spots of ivory-white plaque on the skin. Venous leg ulcers are frequently painful (Hofman et al. 1997).

Assessment and diagnosis

A full medical and nursing patient history and assessment are necessary to identify any factors that may be directly influencing the development of leg ulceration. Nutritional status, mobility, smoking, anaemia, diabetes, the patient's attitude to the ulcer, plus a range of disease processes, may contribute to leg ulceration. It is vital that arterial disease is ruled out at an early stage as the treatment for venous ulceration, compression bandaging, is strongly contraindicated for arterial ulcers.

Identification of the external signs such as ankle flare, lipodermatosclerosis, staining of the skin, eczema, location and characteristics of the ulcer should aid diagnosis.

A differential diagnosis between venous and arterial ulceration can be made using Doppler ultrasonography to assess the blood supply to the leg. The hand-held Doppler probe attached to a recorder directs high-frequency sound waves through the layers of tissue. The sound waves change in frequency when they hit red blood cells and will indicate an obstruction. To establish the adequacy of the peripheral circulation, an ankle–brachial pressure index (ABPI), using Doppler ultrasonography, should be carried out on all patients presenting with lower limb ulceration (Bale, Harding and Leaper 2000). Only when a measurement has been obtained and the cause established can a treatment plan be devised. The following is a step-by-step guide to measuring the ABPI.

The technique of ABPI measurement

- With the patient lying comfortably and as flat as possible place a sphygmomanometer cuff around the calf.
- Apply gel, locate the dorsalis pedis or posterior tibial artery using a hand-held Doppler ultrasound machine.
- Inflate the cuff slowly to the point where the Doppler signal is lost – this is the systolic pressure in the artery.
- The same process is repeated with the brachial artery with a cuff around the upper arm.
- The pressure in the leg is divided by the systolic pressure in the arm to produce the ABPI.
- A pressure index of < 0.8 is suggestive of arterial disease; an APBI of 0.4–0.5 denotes severe arterial disease; ABPI < 0.4 (only 40% of the possible blood flow is managing to get through the artery) denotes critical ischaemia and is a surgical emergency.
- The degenerative arterial effects of diabetes or oedema can skew the accuracy of the reading.

Ankle systolic pressure/Brachial systolic pressure = Ankle–brachial pressure index

Normal ABPI is > 1 in a healthy adult whereas an ABPI of < 0.8 may indicate underlying vascular problems, warranting further diagnostic investigations and precluding compression therapy. Other investigations such as venous duplex scanning, phlebography and venous occlusion plethysmography (VOP) may also be carried out. Venous duplex scanning assesses venous patency and reflux by measuring and recording venous pressures as the veins are released and compressed. Phlebography is a radiological examination of a vein using a contrast medium. VOP measures the rate at which the veins fill or empty to diagnose blood flow distur- bances and occlusions (Collins et al. 2002) using a pressure cuff.

Treatment

When the diagnosis of venous leg ulcer has been confirmed the following are the priorities for care:

- Local wound management: selecting the dressing that is most appropri- ate for managing the exudate levels and to support healing and a dressing that is acceptable to the patient.
- Manage the underlying venous disease, if possible: medication or surgery.
- Control oedema: exercise and elevation.
- Skin care: known sensitizers should be avoided; low allergy emollients such as soft white paraffin/liquid paraffin 50/50 should be applied to keep the skin hydrated and aid removal of skin scales, after washing.
- Limb elevation: the leg should be elevated above the level of the heart, provided that the patient does not have a cardiac or pulmonary condition.
- Compression therapy: multilayer, graduated compression bandages or hosiery to counteract abnormal internal pressures. External bandage pressures of 40 mmHg are needed to manage venous ulceration (Stemmer 1969); training and updating to check proficiency and band- age application pressures should be provided before any nurse is allowed to apply compression bandaging. Short-stretch bandage systems or compression hosiery may be suitable options for those unable to tolerate the multilayer bandage systems. Ideally, compression bandages should be left in place for a week or so; on removal of the bandage, the leg should be washed with warm tap water.
- Prevention of infection: clean wound dressing technique must be employed but there are no known contraindications to the use of tap water for cleansing the wound and leg. Sterile primary dressings are, however, the norm. If strike-through of exudate occurs, the dressings/ bandages should be changed. The wet dressing/bandage will act as an ideal vehicle for the passage of pathogens to the wound. Exudate levels will usually rise if the leg ulcer becomes infected; frequently this will be the first indication of wound infection. Appropriate systemic antibiotic

therapy will be necessary plus the use of silver-containing dressings to treat the infection.

• Patient compliance: many patients have difficulty adjusting to thick, hot, tight bandaging and resent not being able to wear their normal shoes for the sake of a small ulcer. This will, in turn, affect their compliance with treatment. They should be given verbal and written information to help them to understand why the treatment and prevention of recurrence are so important to them.

Regular assessment will include tracings and photographs to monitor healing progress and provide information on which to base treatment decisions. Quality documentation is essential, preferably to include a wound assessment chart. Skin grafting is rarely successful long term as a result of the recurrent nature of venous leg ulcers; alternative wound management therapies are proving to be beneficial. Vacuum-assisted closure, larval therapy, skin substitutes, and grafted skin cells and wound-environment modifying substances are all currently being used to treat leg ulcers successfully.

As the recurrence rate is so high, patients need to be seen at regular intervals to check for deterioration, to ensure that they are wearing their compression hosiery and for general support. 'Leg clubs' have been set up in some parts of the country for these reasons.

Changing patterns of disease

As people age and suffer from conditions such as atherosclerosis, the underlying cause of leg ulceration will alter from venous to mixed venous and arterial disease. This changing pattern should alert the nurse to the necessity for ongoing assessment and revision of treatment plans.

Leg ulcers of vascular origin

Peripheral arterial disease is commonly found in male smokers over the age of 50 years. The male:female ratio is 2:1 between the ages of 50 and 70 years (Dormandy and Ray 1996, Kumar and Clark 2001). Intermittent claudication (leg pain and weakness brought on by exercise and relieved by rest in a patient with arterial disease) (Collins et al. 2002) is present in 5% of the population between the ages of 55 and 75 years and 10% of affected patients have diabetes. Approximately 50 000 people are hospitalized for the treatment of peripheral artery disease each year (Fowkes et al. 1991), consuming a large proportion of the health-care budget.

Peripheral vascular disease is a form of atherosclerosis or hardening of the arteries and is a progressive disease. The result may be arterial blockages affecting arteries in the legs, heart, brain, arms and kidneys, predisposing to gangrene, angina, myocardial infarction or cerebrovascular accident.

Recognized risk factors

Smoking is the most important correctable risk factor for peripheral vascular disease. According to the British Heart Foundation (BHF 1999), approximately 97% of people with peripheral artery disease have smoked for more than 20 years. Other risk factors include hypertension, increased serum cholesterol and triglyceride concentrations, and low high-density-lipoprotein (HDL) cholesterol concentration, i.e. high-fat diet, obesity, lack of exercise, genetic predisposition to high cholesterol levels and diabetes mellitus (Fowkes 1992). Patients who consume excessive amounts of alcohol and/or follow an inappropriate diet may be influenced by or respond to patient education. Arterial ulceration may be preceded by Raynaud's syndrome or sickle-cell anaemia, which are characterized by peripheral ischaemia.

Generally, with an early onset of the disease, symptoms progress more quickly but, in women, it is thought that female hormones offer some protection from arterial disease until the menopause. The picture, however, is changing as a result of the increasing number of women who smoke (BHF 1999). Hasdai et al. (1997) found that a person with no other risk factors has a 30% chance of developing vascular disease just from smoking; smokers had a 44% greater risk of dying from any cause and a 49% greater risk of death from cardiac causes, than those who stopped smoking. However, 63% of patients who underwent bypass surgery continued to smoke. Risk factors are summarized below:

- smoking (past or present)
- high cholesterol
- family history of vascular disease
- sedentary life style
- age
- diabetes mellitus
- being male
- high blood pressure
- atherosclerosis in other areas
- high homocysteine levels
- autoimmune disease.

Peripheral vascular disease is a progressive, inflammatory form of atherosclerosis where fatty degenerative plaques of fat are deposited on the inside walls of the larger arteries and harden (hardening of the arteries). The process continues until the artery walls are no longer elastic and have narrowed. The narrowing of the lumen of the arteries in the limbs results in poor oxygen and nutrient delivery to the areas beyond the narrowing. Cells require a baseline level of oxygen for survival. When this level is reduced, the local tissue dies and, with it, the capacity to regenerate. Thrombosis and total occlusion may occur as a result of advanced disease.

This condition is most likely to occur in the peripheral vessels such as the iliac, femoral and popliteal arteries supplying the legs, the renal arteries supplying the kidneys, the carotid arteries supplying the brain and the subclavian arteries supplying the arms. The arterial changes are exacerbated by hypertension and precede age-related degeneration of the body organs.

Signs and symptoms of peripheral artery disease in the lower limbs

The vessels affected dictate the signs and symptoms. An insufficient supply of oxygen-rich blood results in cramping pain, frequently experienced in the calf muscles, hips, thighs or buttocks on exercise (intermittent claudication). Claudication means limping and was named after the Emperor Claudius who had a limp. The cramping pain and weakness are worse on walking fast, or uphill, disappear on standing still and reappear at set walking distances. Stopping or slowing the rate of walking reduces the demand for oxygen by cells in the muscles. Relief of 'rest pain' at night is achieved by hanging the affected limb down over the side of the bed.

Pain in the lower limb may be confused with diagnoses of sciatica, deep vein thrombosis or muscle injury. If the circulation reduces significantly or the vessel blocks completely, gangrene may result from a thrombus in the artery, leading to amputation of some, or all, of the lower limb.

Other symptoms of peripheral vascular disease in the lower limb include the following:

- absence of pulses
- coldness of the leg and foot
- paleness of the leg and foot, if elevated
- blue/red discoloration of the foot or toes
- fragile, dry, shiny skin
- numbness, pain and/or tingling in the leg, foot or toes
- thickened, brittle toenails
- ulcers that do not heal on the feet, legs and tips of the toes, wherever shoes rub
- ulcers with characteristically smooth, even wound edges with little drainage or oozing, deep, pale pink–grey wound bed
- wound often has dark edges with surrounding pale skin

- infection of the ulcer is a likely complication caused by the compromised vascular supply and location of the wound
- 'Sunset rubra': a phenomenon where the skin of the limb changes to a reddish colour on dependence.

It is frequently at the later stages of the disease that people present for diagnosis because they have managed to adapt their lifestyle to the insidious physiological changes caused by vascular pathology. Untreated, peripheral vascular disease may lead to loss of function, loss of independence and, ultimately, loss of life.

Patients with peripheral vascular disease should be treated in conjunction with a vascular specialist to ensure that the appropriate steps for restoration of adequate blood supply and tissue oxygenation are undertaken in tandem with attempts at wound healing.

Diagnosis

Peripheral vascular disease of the lower extremities, resulting from atherosclerosis, is diagnosed by the type of symptoms present, how the legs appear and the presence or absence of pulses in the feet, legs and groin. The investigation of choice after a comprehensive patient assessment is colour duplex scanning. This will reveal the site of the arterial stenosis causing the symptoms. Arteriography is routinely carried out. Blood lipids should be checked because patients are at risk of stroke and myocardial infarction (BHF 2001).

Treatment

Peripheral vascular disease can be treated with a variety of techniques, including angioplasty, laser treatment and bypass grafts. The simplest of these is balloon angioplasty, in which a catheter is placed in the artery and fed to the area of blockage. A balloon is then inflated to squeeze the fatty blockage against the vessel wall and open the vessel up.

Complications, whether acute, intermediate or chronic, can usually be controlled. Much is being done to prevent and overcome these problems.

Surgical options for arterial disease

With a diagnosis of peripheral vascular disease (PVD), when the pain of atherosclerosis is severe enough to interfere with daily activities, peripheral (leg or arm) bypass surgery may be recommended. Bypass surgery is performed to restore circulation to ischaemic extremities. Surgery involves the creation of a 'detour' past areas where the vessels are blocked. Some types of peripheral bypass are:

- *in situ* bypass
- femoral–popliteal bypass
- femoral–femoral bypass
- aortic–bifemoral bypass.

The type of bypass required is determined by the patient's symptoms, results of investigations and general health status. An incision or multiple incisions may be made from the groin to the knee (or ankle) on the inner leg. With the *in situ* bypass, the saphenous (thigh and calf) vein in the leg is changed into an artery and the blockage or narrowing in the affected artery is bypassed, thereby increasing the blood flow to the foot and leg. In a femoral–popliteal bypass one end of the vein (or a synthetic graft) is attached to the femoral artery in the thigh, above the blockage, whereas the other end is attached to the popliteal artery (knee area) below the blocked area. Blood then flows through the graft and 'bypasses' or detours around the blockage, resulting in improved circulation. In a femoral–femoral bypass, a synthetic graft is attached to the femoral artery of the unaffected leg and tunnelled below the skin of the lower abdomen to the femoral artery of the other leg below the blocked area. Again, the blood flow through the graft renews blood flow. In aortic–bifemoral bypass surgery, a synthetic graft is attached to the aorta and connected to the femoral arteries below the blocked area. Blood flows through the graft, renewing circulation to the legs. A bypass can also be done in the arms to increase blood flow to the fingers.

If the blockage is isolated, a procedure called angioplasty may be an alternative. In this procedure, a balloon-tipped catheter (tube) is passed into the blocked vessel. The balloon is then inflated and the blockage crushed, thereby opening the channel for improved blood flow.

Arterial ulcers

Arterial leg ulcers are the second most common type of leg ulcer after those associated with venous insufficiency. They are the result of underlying arterial disease which reduces the amount of oxygen and nutrients to the cells so that the skin will not function in a normal way. Peripheral artery disease is the prime cause of the ulcer in 10% of all cases (Ruckley et al. 1982, Cornwall et al. 1986, Nelzen et al. 1991). Small and painful ulcers may occur that become chronic, non-healing wounds. Conditions linked with the development of arterial ulcers include the following:

- smoking
- a high-fat/cholesterol diet

- high blood pressure
- stress
- a history of heart disease
- obesity
- diabetes
- rheumatoid arthritis.

It is important to differentiate between ulceration of venous insufficiency and arterial disease and that of mixed arterial and venous origin to ensure that the correct management is instigated. Applying multilayer compression bandaging to treat a venous ulcer is the gold standard, but applying high compression to a vascularly compromised limb will lead to irreversible damage to the tissues. Conversely, if the underlying cause of the venous ulcer, uncontrolled venous hypertension, is left untreated, there is little hope of healing the ulcer although it will not usually be limb or life threatening as with the inappropriate management of the arterial ulcer. A careful medical, nursing and lifestyle assessment is needed before treatment is decided. Table 10.1 compares the signs and symptoms of venous and arterial ulcers (Collier 1996).

Table 10.1 Indications for venous and arterial disease

	Arterial disease	Venous disease
Site	Anywhere, but more common on the foot	Most frequently around the medial malleolus
Pain	Increased at night, with exercise or when the legs are elevated	Dull, aching, relieved by elevation
Skin colour	Legs pale and hairless	Characteristic brown staining above medial malleolus
Oedema	Often seen when legs are dependent	Worse in the evening, reduces with elevation
Toes	Poor capillary refill/cyanosed	
Veins		Often distended
Ulcer	Punched-out, deep with extensive tissue loss	Shallow and flat, high exudate
Eczema		Can be wet, dry, localized or general
Pulses	ABPI < 0.8	ABPI > 0.9
History	Smoking, etc.	Deep vein thrombosis, phlebitis, varicose veins, surgery

Limb preservation is the goal of management by avoiding sepsis, further deterioration of the ulcer and vascular supply and, ultimately, amputation of the limb. Arterial ulcers typically appear on the tips of the toes, between the toes, over the lateral malleolus and phalangeal heads, and lateral aspects of the feet. They often arise after minor trauma with 74% appearing below the ankle level (Baker et al. 1992). Patients will frequently have no recollection of when or how the ulcer occurred.

The lesions are usually well demarcated and deep with a 'punched-out' appearance. The wound bed may be pale and/or filled with necrotic tissue or thick 'tethered slough'; as a result of the depth, there may be bone or tendon visible in the base of the wound. Sensation to light touch and pin prick may be impaired and the wound surrounded by cellulitis.

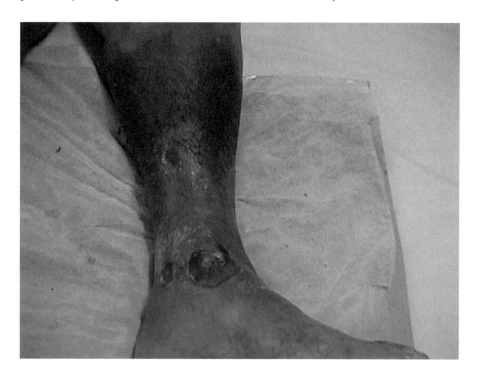

Figure 10.3 Ischaemic leg ulceration (see Plate 15).

Patient assessment

Wound assessment will be the last part of the general patient assessment. It is more important to gather information about the general health, medical problems, lifestyle preferences, dietary habits, level of mobility (especially the walking distance), pain and attitude to illness.

Assessment of the leg will reveal weak or absent peripheral pulses, slow capillary filling, with the leg blanching on elevation and reddening on dependence.

To establish the adequacy of the peripheral circulation, an ABPI, using Doppler ultrasonography, should be carried out on all patients presenting with lower limb ulceration (Bale, Harding and Leaper 2000). Only when a measurement has been obtained and the cause established can a treatment plan be devised.

Accurate, early detection of arterial disease and appropriate management can preserve the limb and the life of the patient (Bale, Harding and Leaper 2000). Management should focus on lifestyle modification, including smoking cessation, weight reduction, if obese, dietary changes, control of hypertension and diabetes (if the patient is diabetic), and a supervised exercise programme to promote the formation of a collateral circulation. Hously (1988) recommends that the patient simply 'stop smoking and get walking'. Drug therapy to prevent arterial occlusion may be prescribed, e.g. aspirin, anticoagulants, statins and anti-claudication therapy.

Critical limb ischaemia is a surgical emergency; amputation is imminent unless the patient is referred rapidly for revascularization and reconstructive surgery. Currently, amputation is performed on patients who have irreversible tissue ischaemia or gangrene caused by vascular disease, uncontrolled diabetes and, more rarely, infection (Ham and Cotton 1991).

Wound management

Wound management should address the following:

- maintain the blood supply to the affected ulcer and limb
- act quickly on detection of deterioration
- reduce the risk of infection by removing necrotic, infected tissue and treating the infection appropriately
- promote healing.

All the modern wound management products can be used to manage arterial wounds but with certain caveats. Maceration of the wound and surrounding skin must be avoided because it will lead to extension of the wound and possible infection resulting from the compromised circulation. Often, gangrenous lesions of the toes are left to dry out without treatment so they will slough off (the black toe found in the bed!). The wound appearance may change rapidly so the nurse must be vigilant and report any seemingly minor changes.

Re-hydration of necrotic tissue with hydrogels may mask the early signs of infection and so they must be used with care (Foster 1999). Hydrocolloids have an effective débriding action but their presence over a wound may also prevent early detection of infection if not changed daily. Hydrofibre dressings are suitable for use in wounds with medium-to-high exudate and may be used for infected wounds if changed daily. As a general rule, vascular wounds should be inspected daily to detect early deterioration (Morgan 2000). The potential is very high for infection with anaerobes in vascular ulcers so dressings containing povidone–iodine are used to keep the bacterial count under control (Finegold 1982). Silver-containing dressings are proving to be effective as local antibacterial agents. In all cases, care must be taken not to allow the dressing to adhere to the already fragile wound bed. Dressings should not be retained with tape or tight bandages; loose bandages or, preferably, tubular bandages should be used to avoid skin trauma.

The selection of dressings will follow on from regular wound assessment, responding to changes to the clinical appearance of the wound and based on the principles of wound management. However, it must be acknowledged that the conservative management of vascular wounds is unpredictable.

Ideally, a dressing will be selected to help heal the ulcer. It should:

• keep the wound moist, clean and warm
• control the amount of leakage from the wound
• control any odour from the wound
• protect the wound from further damage
• be comfortable and not restrict movement
• not cause pain or further damage to the wound when it is removed for re-dressing.

Other effective therapies used to treat vascular wounds include VAC therapy and larval therapy. VAC therapy is used to clear the wound of moist slough, excess exudate, and bacteria and larvae to assist in the removal of slough and necrotic tissue.

The range of therapies grows almost daily but one of the greatest difficulties associated with the care of patients with vascular disease is persuading them to change their lifestyle, in particular smoking cessation. These sentiments are summarized by Goodall (2001) who states that medical management and advice are frequently thwarted or complicated by patient non-compliance with recommended regimens. The severity of the situation is difficult for the patient both to appreciate and to accept that loss of a leg could occur, when all he has is a small ulcer on his toe. All surgical procedures carry risks that must be explained to the patient;

treatment choices have to be balanced against what will happen if, e.g. surgery is not carried out.

The underlying cause of any wound must be identified before attempts at management are made, not least in the case of vascular wounds. Here, there is the possibility of severe irreversible damage to consider, possibly leading to amputation, if the treatment is inappropriate. There is irrefutable evidence that smoking is one of a few correctable, direct causes of peripheral vascular disease but also one of the most difficult to influence in patients with the condition. Globally, emphasis on prevention of peripheral artery disease is vital, with much of the responsibility for disease prevention and prevention of complications being placed in the patient's hands. This is not so easy to achieve, which is why so many more men and women are suffering the effects of peripheral artery disease.

Other causes of leg ulceration include infection, rheumatoid arthritis or other inflammatory diseases (vasculitic ulcers), diabetes, malignancy and trauma (a common occurrence is trauma from supermarket trolleys). Vasculitic ulcers are among the most difficult to heal (Davis et al. 1992) because of the underlying disease.

Diabetic foot ulcers

The overarching key to effective management of patients with diabetic foot ulceration is prevention, early detection and prompt treatment delivered within a multidisciplinary approach (Edmonds et al. 1996). Diabetic foot problems are uncommon before the age of 40 years with the incidence increasing to over 14% in individuals over 80 years of age (Walters et al. 1992). The result is that 45 000 people in the UK have active foot ulceration at one time and approximately 30 000 undergo partial or whole limb amputation each year (Boulton 1994). Patients with diabetes account for the highest number of non-traumatic lower limb amputations (Barnett 1992).

People who have diabetes may present with ulceration associated with neuropathy or ischaemia or a combination of the two pathologies. The most common underlying pathology is peripheral neuropathy (62%) in the lower limb, attributed to nerve damage either caused by an excess of fructose and sorbitol (Watkins et al. 1997) or associated with depleted blood flow as a result of peripheral microvascular disease (Faber et al. 1993). The incidence of foot ulceration increases in line with the duration of the diabetic condition.

The neuropathy may be sensory, motor or autonomic, in isolation or together, accounting for the variety of local symptoms. A further, and serious problem is the presence of infection causing soft tissue necrosis, damage to underlying bone and tendon and increasing the risk of ulceration and amputation.

Diabetic peripheral neuropathy is usually bilateral and symmetrical. The effect of peripheral neuropathy in the lower limb is twofold:

1. Loss of sensation (sensory neuropathy): the patient is unaware of damage being caused by badly fitting shoes, excessive heat or cold, trauma such as that caused when cutting the toenails, treading on sharp or blunt objects, and from over-the-counter corn treatments. Autonomic neuropathy reduces blood flow, causing the skin to be dry; the skin then cracks and fissures and calluses form often masking the full extent of the ulceration. Infection and osteomyelitis will not be readily detected, delaying the necessary débridement and administration of antibiotics.
2. Compromise of the biomechanics of the foot (motor neuropathy): permanent foot deformities such as Charcot's joint (progressive destruction of the joints of the foot that results in bony protrusions in the foot leading to pressure-induced ulceration – Murray and Boulton 1995), claw toes and prominent metatarsal heads may occur as a result of motor neuropathy, muscle atrophy and altered gait.

In contrast with patients who do not have diabetes, where vascular disease affects the larger arteries, the arterioles are initially occluded in patients with diabetes (Wiersema-Bryant and Kraemer 2000). Smoking and ill-fitting footwear are significant risk factors. This may lead to necrosis and gangrene of the toes caused by pressure resulting in occlusion from thrombosis of the artery supplying the toe and the consequent lack of oxygen and nutrients. The effect is that even minor injury may result in a threat to limb and life as a result of infection and septicaemia.

Risk factors for developing diabetic ulceration or gangrene (Connor 1994)

- previous ulceration or gangrene
- increasing age
- peripheral vascular disease
- neuropathy
- structural deformity
- patient non-compliance with management
- duration of diabetes
- male sex
- retinopathy
- nephropathy
- isolation.

Assessment and diagnosis

Any adult presenting with an ulcer of the lower limb must be carefully investigated, diagnosed and treated promptly, particularly those with a pre-existing diagnosis of diabetes. Urinalysis and blood glucose levels should be undertaken to ascertain the glycaemic status of the patient in the case of undiagnosed diabetes. The following must be determined by the health-care professional (Morison and Moffatt 1997):

- the immediate cause of the ulcer, e.g. trauma
- any underlying pathology in the lower limb, e.g. neuropathy
- any local problems at the wound site that may delay healing, e.g. infection
- other more general medical conditions that may delay healing, e.g. anaemia
- current medications
- tobacco and alcohol use
- current glycaemic control
- type and quality of any associated pain
- the patient's social circumstances and the optimum setting for care.

In the person with diabetes, precipitating causes of ulceration may include relatively simple things such as wearing new, ill-fitting shoes, having self or untreated callus, foot injuries, burns from hot bath water, contact with hot sand or hot radiators, using corn plasters, nail infections, heel friction in bed-bound patients or a variety of foot deformities (Watkins 2003).

General assessment will encompass evaluation of all aspects of the patient from mobility to lifestyle. Assessment of the posture, gait, strength, range of motion, balance, reflexes and sensory function will provide a comprehensive view of the patient's physical ability. Assessment of the lower limb pulses will provide information about the integrity of the blood flow to the feet and legs. Assessment of the colour, texture, temperature and appendages of the skin will provide a baseline from which later changes may be compared.

The presence of calluses in certain anatomical locations of the foot should alert the practitioner to the possibility of ulceration. The soles of the feet, tips of the toes, between the toes and the lateral aspect of the foot's plantar surface are common locations for ulceration, and the visual appearance of damage will vary according to the location (Sciarra 2003):

- calluses (pre-wounds)
- blood blisters (haemorrhage beneath a callus)
- erythema, indicating inflammation or infection
- induration (hardened edges)
- skin fissures (portals for bacterial entry)
- dry, scaly skin.

Table 10.2 Clinical features of the neuropathic and ischaemic foot

Neuropathic	Ischaemic (neuroischaemic)
Warm, intact pulses	Pulseless, not warm
Diminished sensation; callus	Usually diminished sensation
Ulceration on tips of toes and plantar surfaces under metatarsal heads	Ulceration often on margins of foot, tips of toes, heels
Sepsis	Sepsis
Local necrosis	Necrosis or gangrene
Oedema	Critical ischaemia (needs urgent referral); foot is pink, painful, pulseless and often cold
Charcot's joints	

Watkins (2003)

Table 10.2 gives the clinical features of neuropathic and ischaemic feet. Diagnostic tests to evaluate pressure, neurological function and vascular perfusion will confirm the diagnosis of diabetic foot ulceration, the mechanism of injury and the prognosis, and guide treatment options. Sophisticated computerized pressure mapping systems are available that will pinpoint high-risk areas of the foot while simple impressions may be obtained using an ink mat to map out the pressure points on the sole of the foot. Other investigations include vibration perception testing with a tuning fork and Semmes–Weinstein monofilament testing for protective sensation. Vascular assessment of the lower limbs through pulse palpation, ABPI, toe pressures and measurement of transcutaneous oxygen levels (TcPo_2 – oxygen saturation of tissues) will be carried out. The ABPI is usually reduced but it should be noted that this index can be inappropriately raised in the person with diabetes as a result of calcification of the arteries.

Diagnostic tests for diabetic foot ulceration

- Vibration perception testing, with a tuning fork or vibration threshold, can be measured using a hand-held biothesiometer. This tests whether the patient has lost protective pain sensation.
- Semmes–Weinstein monofilament testing: this is done with a device with hair-like filaments of different diameters touched to various areas

of the plantar surface of the foot. Areas of thick callus are avoided. Inability to sense the 5.07 monofilament correlates with neuropathy (Wiersema-Bryant and Kraemer 2000).

- ABPI: this is a calculation of arterial efficiency using Doppler ultrasonography. The calculation is made using the highest systolic pressure recorded in the ankle and dividing it by the highest systolic pressure in the arm. The result, in normal arterial flow, should be an ABPI of 1.0 (Collins et al. 2002). In patients with arterial insufficiency, the ABPI would be < 0.8.
- Transcutaneous oxygen levels: a $TcPo_2$ monitor is used to measure oxygen levels in blood externally. Low $TcPo_2$ indicates ischaemia in diabetic foot ulceration (Collins et al. 2002).

Classification of diabetic foot ulcers

After assessment, it is useful to be able to classify the diabetic foot ulcer for future reference. There are several classification systems that classify the ulcer by depth, presence of ischaemia and presence of infection, such as the Wagner (1981) scale (Table 10.3).

Diabetes mellitus impedes healing in several ways that are cumulative in their effects (Davis et al. 1992):

- People with diabetes have a fivefold increase in the risk of wound infection.
- People with diabetes have an impaired inflammatory response resulting in poor quality granulation tissue.
- People with diabetes have atherosclerosis and small vessel disease that impairs blood flow and healing.
- People with diabetes have reduced pain sensation and proprioception – the perception of impulses from the sensory organs (proprioceptors) that give information about the position and movements of the body (Brown 2001).

Table 10.3 Wagner Ulcer Grade Classification System

Grade 0	At-risk foot – pre-ulcerative lesions, healed ulcers, presence of bony deformity
Grade 1	Superficial ulcer, not clinically infected
Grade 2	Deeper ulcer, often infected, no osteomyelitis
Grade 3	Deeper ulcer, abscess formation, osteomyelitis
Grade 4	Localized gangrene (toe, forefoot or heel)
Grade 5	Gangrene of whole foot

Several complications may occur that interfere with healing or herald deterioration. In practice, uncontrolled hyperglycaemia may herald infection and reduce the immune function; poor nutrition and psychosocial factors will impact on positive progress to healing. The signs of infection are often masked as a result of poor immune function, so careful observation of the affected area is important, noting changes in temperature, changes in the appearance of the tissue in the wound and the general state of the patient. Infection may be limb threatening or non-limb threatening. The latter is usually a superficial infection without significant ischaemia and can be treated with antibiotics, sharp débridement and wound cleansing. Limb-threatening infections are established deep in the tissues where there is palpable bone and tissue ischaemia. Surgery to remove the necrotic bone and soft tissue followed by long-term antibiotics and close observation will be necessary to prevent amputation of the limb.

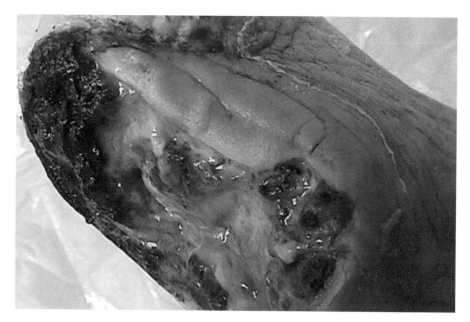

Figure 10.4 Diabetic foot ulcer (see Plate 16).

Management of the patient with diabetic foot ulceration

People with poor glycaemic control are more likely to develop peripheral neuropathy, subsequent foot ulceration and impaired healing (Boulton 1996, Mayfield et al. 1998). It is, therefore, essential to promote normoglycaemia as far as possible. Deteriorating sight associated with diabetic retinopathy combined with neuropathy will impede early detection of ulceration because patients will be unable to feel or see damage to their feet – a magnifying glass may help.

Callus formation is a protective mechanism to external trauma that may disguise an ulcerated area. Any external trauma must be removed and patients educated to protect their feet from further damage. The patient should be advised to wear well-fitting shoes, not walk barefoot, to check the inside of footwear and socks for sharp material, check the temperature of bath water with the hand, and avoid using hot water bottles and foot spas. Temporary casts or special boots/sandals may be used until the ulcer heals and the patient can then obtain specialized footwear that redistributes the pressure away from the bony prominences. The skin must also be kept in good condition by regularly moisturizing around the wound area with emollients.

Regular screening of the feet, as part of a diabetic screening programme, should be undertaken by the community or practice nurse, documented and shared with the local diabetes team. Patients with hard skin or corns must be dissuaded from using over-the-counter caustic remedies (corn plasters contain chemicals that can damage the healthy tissues), and be assessed and treated by the podiatrist regularly. Callus should be removed by a state-registered chiropodist or podiatrist to prevent build-up with the risk of subsequent ulceration, infection and increased local foot pressures. Débridement should extend to the base of the ulcer to allow the wound to granulate (Jones 1998).

Dressing choice should be based on the principles of wound healing, which are the same as for any wound type except that consideration must be given to the type of ulcer, its location and whether special footwear or casts are being worn (Jones and Gill 1998). Appropriate systemic antibiotic therapy will be indicated at different times to treat aerobic and anaerobic infection during the time taken to heal the ulcer. Casts should not be used if the ulcer is infected and producing a large volume of exudate because they will need regular inspection, cleaning and dressing change.

If the wound bed is dry and necrotic, it should be gently re-hydrated and de-sloughed using hydrogels or hydrocolloid dressings, avoiding maceration. The removal of necrotic material reduces the risk of infection and expedites wound healing (Sciarra 2003). Surgical débridement is necessary for deep or spreading tissue infection or osteomyelitis. If the exudate levels are high, then an alginate, hydrofibre or foam dressing should be used. Iodine-impregnated dressings are commonly used to reduce the bacterial count in the wound. Newer, slow-release silver dressings are proving to be useful in inhibiting bacterial growth. Documentation must be concise and timely with photographs and linear measurements, rather than tracings, used to track healing progress because there will usually be little noticeable change in the size of the wound (Dealey 2000). Research is ongoing into the use of topically applied growth factors but their therapeutic effect is dependent on an adequate vascular supply and wound bed preparation. Living skin equivalents, e.g. Dermagraft, are also being researched as interactive wound coverings to enhance healing rates (Grey et al. 1998b).

General guidance for prevention of diabetic foot ulceration

The most important factor influencing the prevention and development of diabetic complications is persuading patients to take responsibility for their own health. Patients and their carers should be educated about the relevant risk factors and how to eliminate or manage the risks. Good foot care is vital to prevent ulceration and should include daily skin inspection, careful washing and drying, toenail care, appropriate footwear and exercise.

Fungating wounds

A fungating tumour is defined as tumour infiltration into the skin forming a raised exuding fungus-like growth, which grows rapidly (Collins et al. 2002). They are particularly difficult wounds to manage, distressing for the nurse and patient, and consume a large amount of nursing time. They are found in adult patients across the whole age range. Again, there is no standard treatment; symptomatic management of excess exudate, bleeding, malodour and discomfort is a priority for the patient often at different stages of the disease process. Little is known about the prevalence of fungating wounds and published data on their aetiology and management are lacking (Sims and Fitzgerald 1985, Grocott 1995b).

Fungating wounds may arise from primary, secondary or recurrent malignancy so, for many patients, treatment will be palliative. Approximately 5–10% of patients with metastatic cancer will develop a fungating wound (Haisfield-Wolfe and Rund 1997). Fungating lesions of the breast (62%) are most common (Thomas 1992), but other body areas such as the head and neck (24%) (Thomas 1992), abdomen, sacrum, shoulder and mid-thigh have been reported. Tumours associated with fungating wounds include squamous cell and basal cell carcinoma and malignant melanoma (Naylor 2001). The absence of pain in the early stages of tumour development contributes to the delayed presentation to the general practitioner for treatment.

Aetiology

The fungating lesion develops in a complex manner, as a result of infiltration of the epithelium by cancerous cells through the processes of

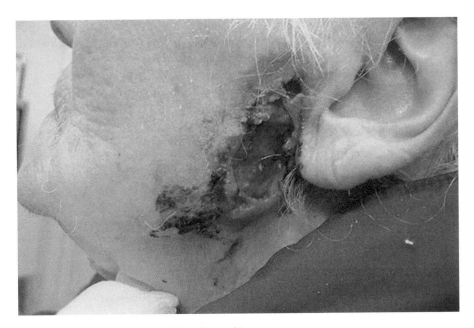

Figure 10.5 Fungating wound (see Plate 17).

ulceration and proliferation. The events that lead to the development of a fungating lesion involve blood haemostasis, and lymph, interstitial and cellular environments (Bridel-Nixon 1997b). Distortion of the vasculature and local tissue destruction impede blood flow, resulting in the formation of necrotic tissue which provides an ideal environment for aerobic and anaerobic bacteria to flourish. Malodour is a common complication resulting from the production of volatile fatty acids as metabolic waste (Mortimer 1993). Localized infection will increase exudate levels and malodour.

Signs and symptoms

Initially, fungating wounds present as discrete non-tender nodules coloured black/brown, pink, violet or blue which, as they increase in size, may develop into a raised nodular lesion or an ulcerating lesion with a characteristic 'lip' around the edge (Moody and Grocott 1993). With the extension of tissue necrosis and disruption of skin capillaries come tissue hypoxia and skin necrosis, and the constant possibility of sinus or fistula development. The wound tissue is friable and bleeds easily as a result of decreased platelet function and pressure on the tissues from tumour infiltration (Haisfield-Wolfe and Rund 1997).

Each fungating wound is unique, possessing different characteristics and symptoms, and so it will require individualized management according to wound assessment findings. The patient will often direct the priorities of management based on the symptoms that they find most troublesome, e.g. if the patient finds the odour particularly offensive that is the priority, particularly if it is interfering with activities of daily living such as eating or socializing. The management of a patient with a fungating wound will usually be palliative so all efforts to preserve their dignity, sense of well-being and quality of life must be addressed.

Treatment

Palliative radiotherapy may be offered to the patient to alleviate some of the symptoms and reduce the size of the tumour.

Wound management

The wound should be assessed according to the guidance given in Chapter 7, as for any wound but with particular attention to the following:

- the presence of slough, necrotic or infected tissue
- excessive exudate
- malodour
- the position of the wound especially when it has spread to areas of the body that are difficult to dress, e.g. the axilla and/or eroded axillary lymph nodes, causing leakage of lymphatic fluid
- bleeding
- lymphoedema (Dealey 2000)
- bulky dressings and inconvenience
- fear – as an obvious reminder of malignancy (Bridel-Nixon 1997b).

Dressings for fungating wounds

Exudate management

There is a wide range of absorbent dressings suitable for managing excessive wound exudates, including hydrocellular foam, alginate, hydrofibre dressings and, more recently, capillary action dressings. These products are designed to provide comfort and dryness, to reduce leakage and soiling of clothes, and to promote confidence using discrete, non-bulky, well-fitting dressings. Important factors to consider are:

- prevention of strike-through to reduce the frequency of dressing changes and malodour
- maintenance of a moist wound environment to minimize pain and bleeding during dressing change

- the size and bulkiness of the dressing which will affect movement and body image.

There are several dressing combinations that include a non-adherent primary dressing, odour-reducing medication, absorbent dressing, pads and secondary retention dressing. The non-adherent primary dressing is vital to prevent trauma to the already friable tissue during dressing removal and to maintain a moist wound–dressing interface. Mepitel, Urgotul or similar products will provide the necessary conditions.

Odour control

Metronidazole gel is frequently used to reduce the bacterial count at the wound site effectively to minimize odour. Débridement is recommended using a hydrogel to rid the wound of necrotic tissue, and to reduce the risk of anaerobic infection, increased exudate and odour.

Charcoal dressings have been used extensively in the past for their odour-absorbing properties. Silver-containing dressings are now available as hydrocolloid, foam and wound contact layers, which are proving to be beneficial in reducing the inflammation and odour, and therefore exudate, in fungating wounds.

Managing bleeding

Capillary bleeding can alarm both the patient and the nurse and is the result of local erosion of capillaries by the tumour. Dressings must not be allowed to adhere to the wound bed and cause trauma and bleeding on removal. Adrenaline (epinephrine) may be applied directly to the bleeding points in the wound but should be used with caution under medical supervision. Some alginate dressings have haemostatic properties, which will be useful for oozing; it may be necessary carefully to irrigate or soak the dressing off with saline to prevent further bleeding. The patient's blood should be checked to ensure that anaemia is not occurring as a result of bleeding from the wound.

The size, bulk, location and retention of the dressing may cause inconvenience and low self-esteem. Fungating wounds often present in areas of the body that are difficult both to dress and to achieve retention of the dressing for an appreciable period of time, e.g. a fungating breast wound may present on the upper chest wall, and extend into the axilla, restricting movement as a result of padding and fear of dislodging the dressing. The trick is to be creative with products and devices designed to manage the wound; mixing dressing products is acceptable, provided that sound rationale is behind the choice of products (Benbow 2000). Sealing the dressing well will reduce the odour and contain the exudates, allowing fewer dressing changes as a result of odour and leakage.

Care of the surrounding skin

As a result of frequent dressing changes, high exudate levels and the overall unpredictability of the fungating wound, it is wise to protect the surrounding skin from an early stage of management. Non-sting barrier products such as Cavilon are rapidly becoming a mainstay in skin protection of all kinds. The cream is suitable for protecting intact skin where damage is expected, with the barrier film more suitable for superficially damaged skin. The skin surrounding a wound must be kept clean and dry at all times, both to protect against invasion of the wound by skin bacteria and for aesthetic reasons.

The skin must also be protected from damage caused by radiation therapy and simple skin tapes, which should never be attached to fragile skin. Tubular bandages, net and gauze are more appropriate if needed for dressing retention. Patients with cancer-associated lymphoedema will require more specialized management of the condition and its effects on the skin, i.e. to massage and moisturize the swollen skin and prevent cracking in the skinfolds and compression to reduce the swelling.

Fistulae and sinuses

A fistula is a passage that has formed between two organs, e.g. the bowel and the skin (Collins et al. 2002). The incidence, morbidity and mortality of enterocutaneous fistulae are unknown as a result of the variance in the number of organs involved (Jeter et al. 1990, Rolstad and Bryant 2000). The output from a fistula may comprise blood, digestive contents, bile, faeces or urine. Fistulae may develop spontaneously or following surgery (90%) (Rinsema 1992) and may connect the rectum with the vagina (rectovaginal), from the bile duct to the skin (biliary), or from the bowel to the skin surface. Fistulae may be single tract or complicated with multiple tracts (Pringle 1995). Fistula development may be associated with various disease processes such as malignancy and inflammatory bowel disease, and may be planned or spontaneous. The underlying cause will determine the outcome of treatment, e.g. if the fistula is associated with malignancy, it is unlikely to close, but, if it is associated with Crohn's disease, there is the likelihood of closure as exacerbation of the disease abates.

Management

There is little research evidence on which to base treatment decisions; most treatment is experiential relating to the management of fistulae. The three main considerations will be the care of the surrounding skin, manipulation

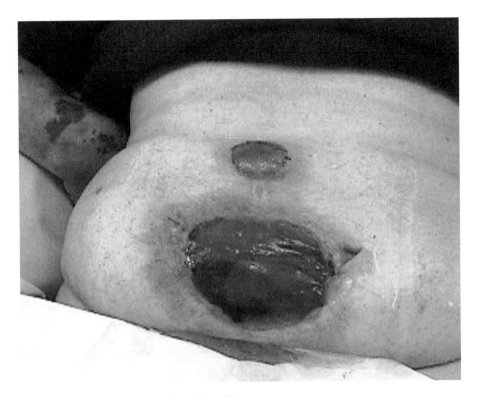

Figure 10.6 Intestinal fistula (see Plate 18).

of the conditions that will aid closure and surgical correction (Borwell 1994). The difficulties likely to be encountered relate to the loss of large volumes of fluid and electrolytes, their replacement and the corrosive nature of the effluent if it comes into contact with skin. Dietetic assessment is vital if fluid loss is excessive, followed by appropriate nutritional support orally, parenterally or intravenously. Management of the consistency and volume of the effluent may also be necessary by adding fibre to the diet if appropriate. Medication to reduce the production of gastric secretions may also be considered to reduce the volume of effluent. Other important considerations include maintaining patient mobility, odour control, patient comfort and acceptability, accurate measurement of effluent and cost-containment (Cobb and Knaggs 2003).

Regular assessment of the wound/fistula is essential to identify changes in the wound exudate – consistency, volume, characteristics and skin condition. The unpredictability associated with the management of fistulae will direct patient and wound management.

Generally, neither traditional nor modern wound management products have the capacity to contain the vast amounts of effluent from a fistula. If the output is over 100 ml/24 h, a wound management bag is recommended (Black 1995). The wound management bag may be single use, disposable or drainable to extend its wear time and reduce the inconvenience to the patient during too-frequent bag changes. Ultimately, in the event of non-healing in a patient with good life expectancy, surgery may be carried out to lay open the fistula and encourage healing by secondary intention. Corrosive effluent leakage on to the skin can result in severe excoriation which is painful and difficult to treat because of its proximity to the fistula. Skin protection should be instigated as early as possible and comprises a combination of filler paste, ostomy seals and hydrocolloid protective skin wafers. Debris left on the skin from previous devices should be carefully removed before reapplication of a new device/dressing and the surrounding skin treated with a non-sting barrier film. Security of adherence of the device will prevent leakage and maintain good patient morale and comfort. The use of topical negative pressure (VAC therapy) was contraindicated for enterocutaneous fistulae, but it was found in a recent study that it can control effluent output effectively and does not preclude spontaneous closure of the fistula (Nienhuijs et al. 2003).

Sinuses

A sinus is a blind-ended, epithelial cell-lined tube from the outside of the body to inside, forming a sinusoidal cavity, sometimes leading to specific structures such as a bursa. The origin of a sinus may be an abscess that has used the track to evacuate pus or a foreign body deep in the tissues, such as a suture or one that becomes a focus for infection (Collins et al. 2002), osteomyelitis or necrotic tissue. If a sinus tract is present, it is important to ascertain its extent, direction and duration. Sinuses may become chronic if symptoms persist over several months without signs of abating. The underlying cause must be identified and, if possible, removed surgically, leaving the wound to heal by either primary closure or secondary intention.

Pilonidal sinus is the only type of sinus that has been considered in the literature. This usually occurs in men aged between 20 and 30 years in the sacrococcygeal area as a result of keratin plugs penetrating the skin, creating a cavity that encourages the entry of debris, including hair (Bridel-Nixon 1997b). A foreign body reaction occurs with epithelialization of the cavity and formation of a sinus. Pain, discomfort and discharge are the most frequently reported symptoms, with many developing a pilonidal abscess that needs antibiotic therapy and surgery. There are disagreements about whether the first-line treatment should be surgery or conservative management and prevention. Preventive measures such as shaving the area, good hygiene and patient education are advocated and the condition appears to be self-limiting. Surgical management, by excision and primary closure, is advocated to reduce time lost from work, time spent in hospital and time to heal; however, there are various forms of surgery carried out. There appears to be little consensus generally about best practice in the management of pilonidal sinuses. Factors to consider when deciding patient management for pilonidal sinus include:

- patient history
- presenting symptoms (abscess or sinus)
- employment status
- patient choice
- cost
- local expertise.

Both fistulae and sinuses are abnormal structures that develop as a result of distortion in the normal structure of the body. They can be disfiguring, inconvenient and lead to psychosocial problems in patients as a result of anxiety about odour and leakage. They are frequently long-term problems during which time patients may become depressed and concerned about the outcome of the problem. These are complex wounds that require expert attention, high-quality assessment and management.

Conclusion

This chapter has briefly outlined some of the more common chronic wounds encountered by nurses, their aetiology, clinical presentation, prevention and management.

Student exercises

- What measures would you instigate to prevent a patient developing a pressure ulcer from first contact either in the community or in hospital?
- How would you attempt to improve compliance in a patient newly diagnosed with type 2 diabetes?
- How would you reassure a patient with a fungating malignant wound?

CHAPTER ELEVEN

Classification and treatment of different wound types: acute wounds

Minor injuries

This chapter describes the more common minor injuries encountered in an accident and emergency department (A&E), their assessment and management. The majority of patients presenting to A&E with minor wounds usually heal without incident or complication. A wound is a break in the epidermis or dermis that can be related to trauma or pathological changes within the skin or body (Collins et al. 2002) associated with a loss of substance (Lippert 1999).

Wounds account for approximately 25–30% of the total workload of an A&E (Wardrope and Smith 1992) with lacerations from blunt trauma being the most common. Cuts, bruises, abrasions and burns are also common. Traumatic wounds can range from minor cuts to extensive burns or crushing injuries. The management of major traumatic injuries is beyond the remit of this book and will normally require specialist surgical intervention. Minor wounds such as lacerations are, however, managed by nurses on a regular basis and may be the result of accidents at work, in the home or during recreational activities. Road traffic accidents, physical assault, animal bites and self-inflicted injuries account for a large number of admissions to A&E.

Although the wound may be minor to the nurse, it may present major anxieties, pain, shock and suffering to the patient. Patient assessment should accurately confirm the minor nature of the wound and absence of potential complications such as airway obstruction, hypovolaemic shock or haemorrhage. Late medical or medico-legal problems may result from incomplete assessment that later reveals undetected fractures, foreign bodies or nerve injury. A history of how, when and where the patient sustained the wound should be complemented by a medical history including any medications that the patient is currently taking. The medical history may contain factors that will affect healing or the choice of management.

In A&E, patients with minor injuries are triaged based on the severity of their injury. There are three key elements to consider at triage:

1. accurate description of the wound
2. documentation of the mechanism of injury, tetanus immunization status, current medication and known allergies
3. first aid measures for haemostasis, proper cleansing and temporary closure of open wounds, which will lengthen the time for definitive management.

Types of traumatic wounds

- A cut is a breach or tear in the skin usually caused by a sharp object such as metal, glass or wood. Cuts characteristically have straight, well-defined wound edges with little soft tissue bruising or damage. With little tissue loss, cuts will heal without any problems if sutured and covered with a simple non-adherent dressing and tape depending on their location.
- Lacerations are breaches or splits in the skin caused by a blunt instrument or force, e.g. the result of a fall, crushing injury or blow with a blunt instrument over a bony prominence. The wound edges are characteristically jagged and irregular, with evidence of tearing of the subcutaneous or deeper tissues and associated bruising. The severity of the laceration will depend on its cause, size, depth and location.
- Contusions or bruises occur as a result of the rupture of subcutaneous or deeper blood vessels following an impact (Mant 1985). The skin may be intact, abraded or lacerated, spreading to occupy a greater surface area than the instrument that caused them. The fluid element of the bruise will be absorbed back into the blood stream. Gripping injuries may produce distinguishable discrete bruising or erythematosus weals as in cases of child abuse.
- Abrasions are partial-thickness (superficial) injuries often caused by friction or shearing forces between the skin and the blunt object. Abrasions may scab over and heal without scarring.
- Skin tears are specific types of laceration that mostly affect older people with fragile skin as a result of the ageing process, medications or dermatological conditions. Frequently the degree of trauma is minimal and the force exerted is one of a shearing or frictional nature that separates the layers of skin. In the case of the epidermis separating from the dermis, this would produce a partial-thickness wound; if the dermis/ epidermis separates from the underlying tissues a full-thickness wound results. Skin tears can be prevented in the main by careful handling of the elderly person when helping to move or re-position them. Skin tears

can be problematic in areas such as the shin because the vascular supply is poor and prolonged healing should be expected. The choice of primary and secondary dressings should take into account the fragile nature of the patient's skin and be totally non-adherent to the wound bed; ideally, secondary dressings should not be attached to the skin surrounding the wound. Extensible and tubular bandages should be selected in preference to adhesive secondary dressings/retention products to reduce the risk of further skin damage.

- Bites: the most important issue is the source of the bite – was it a dog, cat, spider, snake, human? Knowing the cause of the bite will guide the team towards deciding what toxins or bacteria are present and what type of tissue trauma should be expected. The brown recluse spider, native to parts of the USA, has the capacity to inflict necrotizing wounds on unfortunate individuals. Dogs have large teeth that are capable of causing tearing and crushing injuries; lacerations occur in 30–45% of cases, puncture wounds in 13–34% and superficial abrasions in 30–43% (Dire 1992). Cats have fine, sharp teeth and, despite a weaker bite, are capable of penetrating bone and joint capsules (Smith et al. 2000). Puncture wounds occur in 57–86% of cases, lacerations in 5–17% and superficial abrasions in 9–25% (Dire 1992). Most adult human bites (60–75%) occur on the hand. Clenched fist injury (caused by hitting another person's teeth with a clenched fist) is common, and is particularly prone to infection (Monteiro 1995, Smith et al. 2000). Careful wound cleansing, removal of foreign material and suturing, if appropriate, should be carried out. If the wound is heavily contaminated with debris, it may be left open for a few days dressed with a non-adherent dressing, under antibiotic cover, and then sutured.

Healing considerations in minor wounds

- Anatomical site: vascularity at the site plays a major role, e.g. pre-tibial lacerations heal slowly as a result of poor blood supply; head and neck wounds heal more quickly because of the rich vascular supply; people with peripheral vascular disease will heal more slowly than those without. Movement over a joint will also delay healing.
- Delay in management: wounds will be exposed to a mixture of pathogens until they have been treated which may lead to contamination, infection and subsequently delayed healing.
- Wound configuration: simple, tidy uncomplicated wounds heal faster than jagged wounds with large areas of skin loss and/or devitalized tissue.
- Mechanism of injury: incised wounds heal faster than lacerations from blunt trauma.

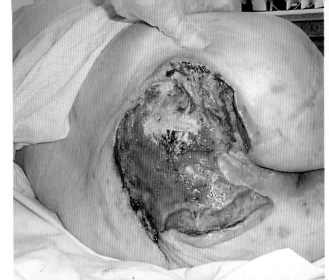

Plate 13 Sacral pressure ulceration.

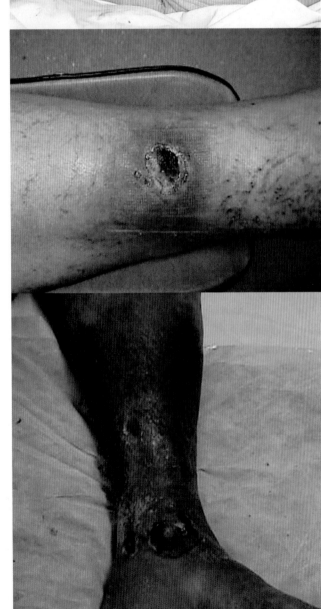

Plate 14 Venous leg ulcer.

Plate 15 Ischaemic leg ulceration.

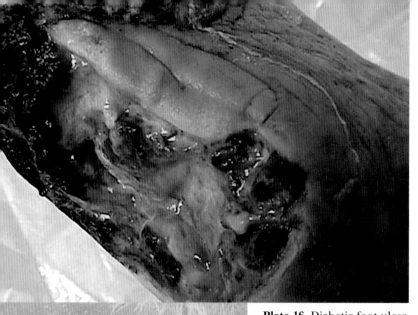

Plate 16 Diabetic foot ulcer.

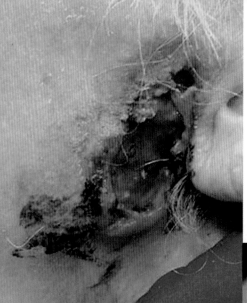

Plate 17 Fungating wound.

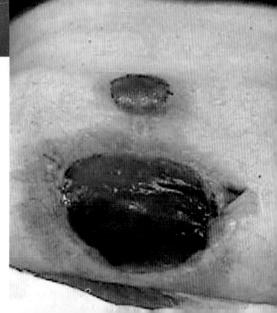

Plate 18 Intestinal fistula.

- General health and nutrition considerations: wound healing is impeded by deficiency of vitamin C and zinc; older patients may have cardiovascular or endocrine disease (diabetes mellitus) which will also interfere with healing; it has long been recognized that taking long-term steroid medication weakens and causes changes to the skin and influences healing rates.

Treatment of minor injuries

Cleansing

Wound cleansing is vital to remove debris, potential contaminants, remnants of previous dressings and devitalized tissue. Irrigation at < 8 lb/in^2 (psi) of pressure with sterile 0.9% saline or tap water (of drinking quality) is the preferred method (Moscati et al. 1998). Traditional antiseptic solutions are no longer recommended for use in wound cleansing because they need extended contact with the wound surface to exert any antibacterial effect (Thomas 1990). Chlorhexidine, cetrimide, EUSOL, proflavine and potassium permanganate have no real benefits to offer in wound care (Dealey 2000).

Toxicity associated with antiseptics has been identified in laboratory tests on cultured keratinocytes (Tatnall et al. 1990). Hydrogen peroxide has been used effectively to remove debris and slough from wounds mechanically; however, even in weak solution it was shown to inhibit keratinocyte migration and proliferation necessary for healing (O'Toole et al. 1997). Air embolism has been reported in connection with hydrogen peroxide irrigation, which should not be carried out on cavity wounds (Sleigh and Linter 1985). Prolonged antiseptic action is achieved by using hydrogen peroxide in a 1.5% cream form. Hydrogen peroxide, if still used, should be limited in the number of applications and the wound should be irrigated with saline afterwards (Dealey 2000).

Iodine, however, continues to be a popular choice of broad-spectrum antiseptic used in A&E departments and vascular surgery wards, in several forms. Inadine dressing is a topical antimicrobial wound dressing impregnated with an ointment containing 10% povidone–iodine, providing a sustained release of iodine. Inadine is commonly used to treat minor injuries in A&E; the dressing changes colour from orange to white when the iodine is no longer active. Inadine tends, however, to dry out quickly and can adhere to the wound and cause trauma on removal. Povidone–iodine is the aqueous solution most used in wound care as a skin disinfectant and to clean infected wounds such as those that are infected with methicillin-resistant *Staphylococcus aureus* (MRSA) or before surgery to reduce the bacterial count.

Iodine is used despite several associated drawbacks:

- cytotoxic to fibroblasts except in very dilute concentrations
- should not be used in patients with thyroid disease or sensitivity
- no more effective than sterile saline in preventing infection (Becker 1986)
- lowers the tensile strength of the wound (Lineaweaver et al. 1985).

Although the use of iodine is prevalent, more research is needed to justify its continued use. Silver-containing dressings are, in many cases, promoted for use in the pre-infected wound or those wounds in patients who are at high risk for infection. The extra cost of these dressings may preclude their use in this area.

Closure

Sutures, fabric skin closures and tissue adhesives are used depending on the severity, location and history of the wound and, where necessary, covered with a low-adherent or non-adherent dressing.

Dressings

There is a range of modern wound management products available to dress traumatic wounds, with the choice depending on the type of wound, its location, the presence or risk of infection, the amount of exudate (Thomas 1997a) and social reasons. Most minor traumatic wounds produce little exudate so hydrocolloid dressings or semi-permeable film dressings may be suitable. Non-adherent dressings should be a priority for wounds in which dried exudate or blood may cause trauma and pain on removal such as fingertip injuries, lacerations and abrasions. Tulle dressings such as Jelonet should be avoided because of their propensity to dry out and stick to the wound bed, and the likelihood of ingrowth of granulation tissue into the open weave of the dressing will cause both trauma and pain on dressing removal. Antibiotics for topical use are available but are potentially hazardous and not always absorbed into the wound. However, mupirocin is one antibiotic that is widely used to treat wounds that are infected with methicillin-resistant *Staphylococcus aureus* (MRSA). There is also the potential for sensitization and resistance associated with generalized inappropriate antibiotic use.

Patient education and self-care

Patients should be given information orally about their injury, its implications and expected outcome. They should also be informed about the treatment, i.e. the type of dressing, its properties, e.g. whether it is water resistant, how it performs, its wear time and any changes in structure, colour or consistency that might be expected while it is in place. Easy-to-understand, relevant written information in the form of an information leaflet should be given to back up oral information and clarify any queries that the patient may have. Basic practical safety instructions such as not wetting a cotton dressing and not smoking while wearing an inflammable dressing should be emphasized.

Comprehensive assessment and accurate documentation are particularly important in the A&E setting to protect the patient and the health-care professional. Medicolegal issues may arise long after the wound has healed, possibly because the patient has been left with a residual disability from their injury which they feel should have been prevented. The written documentation is the only reliable source of information to defend the actions of health-care staff, so it must be clear, concise, accurate and contemporaneous.

Surgical wounds

An acute surgical wound is a healthy, uncomplicated, intentional breach in the normal skin barrier as a result of surgery. In otherwise healthy individuals, with no or minimal tissue loss, and with the right management, the wound will heal without adverse incident by primary intention. Significant factors that may impede healing are advancing age, poor nutritional status, oxygenation, traumatic tissue handling and general health status before surgery. Age is an important factor for both the very young and the very old patient. In the pre-term infant the immune and other body systems may not be well developed, increasing the risk of infection before, during and after surgery. Various systemic disease processes, and skin and tissue changes caused by the ageing process, which impair the immune system, may affect the elderly patient, leading to delayed healing and an increase in the risk of infection.

Nutritional deficits in any post-surgical patient must be addressed promptly because healing depends on adequate supplies of the range of nutrients. After surgery, the body is depleted of nutrients which must be replaced to maintain homoeostasis and provide the right conditions for healing, i.e. the delivery of adequate supplies of nutrients to the wound site.

The presence of excess adipose tissue (fat) in a person does not always imply that the person is well nourished. As the amount of adipose tissue increases, so the vascularity of the skin decreases, because adipose tissue is not well vascularized, which, in turn, will lead to problems with healing.

The majority of patients undergoing both elective and emergency surgery are elderly with pre-existing illnesses or infections that may delay or complicate healing. The following will be of particular interest:

- conditions that reduce the flow of blood to the injured area, e.g. coronary artery and peripheral vascular disease
- cancer; the patient may be taking immunosuppressive medications and require higher doses of analgesia
- diabetes mellitus is known to interfere with healing in many ways and adversely affect wound healing
- conditions that interfere with the local delivery of oxygen to the wound site, e.g. anaemia, atherosclerosis.

Surgical wounds may be described as follows:

- clean, i.e. the gastrointestinal, genitourinary or respiratory tracts are not opened, e.g. varicose veins
- clean contaminated, i.e. a tract may be opened, but there is minimal spillage of contents, e.g. elective cholecystectomy
- contaminated, i.e. acute inflammation without pus or when there is gross spillage from an opened tract, e.g. elective colorectal surgery with poor bowel preparation
- dirty, i.e. pus is encountered or a perforated tract is found, e.g. perforated duodenal ulcer with peritonitis (Coull 2003).

Wound closure

The surgeon will decide on the most appropriate method of wound closure based on the severity of the wound and the patient history. The most commonly used methods of closure are with the use of:

- suture materials
- skin staples or clips
- adhesive skin closures
- skin closure adhesive.

Suture materials

A suture is a natural or synthetic material passed through each side of the wound and securely knotted. Non-absorbable sutures are used to close the skin surface wound to provide strength and immobility and to minimize tissue irritation. Subcuticular sutures may be used to minimize scarring. Examples of non-absorbable sutures include silk, Dacron, cotton and stainless steel. Absorbable sutures are used when removal is not required or desirable in the deeper tissues; these may be chromic catgut (longer absorption time), plain catgut (absorbed faster) and synthetic materials, e.g. polyglycolic acid, which are less irritant, stronger and more durable than catgut. Depending on the location of the wound, extent of surgery, the surgeon and any previous complications, skin sutures may be removed between 5 and 10 days postoperatively. Non-absorbable, continuous sutures should be removed by supporting the wound with one hand, and gently pulling the suture through with the other hand along the line of the wound.

Skin staples and clips

The technique of skin stapling was pioneered in Russia, and later spread to the West through 'informal' channels. The pioneers had huge instruments that took a long time to load with staples, e.g. Hultl's stapler of 1908 weighed 8 lb (3.6 kg), and required 2 hours to assemble and load. In the earliest days, almost everything was tried to get consistent staple lines, including the use of common office staples. Soon, however, titanium came to be accepted as the ideal staple material for surgery. Surgical staplers are commercially manufactured today either in stainless steel, to be cleaned and re-used, or in plastic for single use. The biggest improvement over the old hand-built staplers is in the staples themselves. Early staples were hand formed and inconsistent; now they are supplied pre-loaded in cartridges, and the better staplers have features such as overlapping staple lines, B-shaped staples (which do not crush tissue) and optional knife blades, so that the blade that passes through contaminated and possibly cancerous tissue is used only once, then discarded. The result is a tissue join that is patent, consistent and stable over time. Benefits to the patient include dramatically reduced rates of infection and faster recovery times.

Staples can also be used in minimally invasive or 'keyhole' surgery, where accurate suturing is very challenging, or even for simple skin repairs such as to deep scalp lacerations. The staples/clips are removed using a disposable removal device and by inserting under the clip/staple and closing the remover over the top. This will cause the clip/staple to bend in the middle and release the sides from the skin.

Adhesive skin closure strips (Steri-Strips) or butterfly closures

These may be used for smaller wounds with little drainage or after suture or clip removal for wound support. Space should always be left between the skin closures to allow for drainage.

Skin closure adhesive

This is widely used among plastic surgeons and in A&E departments with good results (Ellis and Shaikh 1990, Saltz and Zamora 1998). When not used in high-tension areas, such as a joint, the use of skin closure glue is as effective as conventional suturing in terms of both infection rate and cosmetic appearance after surgery when applied by a suitably trained person (Simon et al. 1997). Within the plastic surgery field, surgical glue has been used widely with good effects, because it appears to reduce the bruising, oedema and bleeding associated with this type of surgery (Ellis and Shaikh 1990, Saltz and Zamora 1998).

This technology allows surgeons to close patients' skin without using sutures, the removal of which can be painful and traumatic. This is especially useful in the case of children, or when small-calibre sutures must be removed from sensitive areas of the face (such as the nose, eyelids or lips). New technology in surgical adhesives could provide all patients with the option of suture-less skin closure. The ideal adhesive would:

• be safe for topical application
• be easy to apply
• polymerize rapidly
• support the approximated skin edges and maintain the skin-edge eversion necessary for maximum wound healing and acceptable cosmesis
• eliminate the need for suture removal.

The main advantages associated with non-invasive methods of skin closure are reduced pain, no follow-up for suture removal, and less stress and anxiety particularly in children. Ranaboldo and Rowe-Jones (1992) found that laparotomy wounds closed with staples were more painful than wounds closed with subcuticular polydioxanone sutures.

Dressings for surgical wounds

The purpose of applying a dressing to a surgically created wound is to protect it against pathogens, to protect the skin from exudate and for aesthetic reasons. Within 48 hours, the wound is sealed with fibrin and so impervious to bacteria (Dealey 2000); however, patients will often prefer to have their wound dressed to prevent sutures, clips, etc. from snagging on their clothes. The type of surgery and subsequent volume of drainage will guide the choice of dressing; wounds with minimal exudate will need only a non-adherent contact layer and tape. Wounds with higher levels of exudate will need a more absorbent primary and possibly secondary dressing to protect the surrounding skin.

Patient education is important both to reduce the risk of wound infection and to protect the new wound. The patient must be advised not to interfere with the dressing, be taught good hand-washing technique and be encouraged to eat a suitably nourishing diet to support healing.

Most surgical wounds will heal without incident by primary intention but there are certain complications that the health-care professional must know about:

- wound infection caused by competition for nutrients and oxygen between the tissues and bacteria in the wound, preventing healing
- wound dehiscence: spontaneous separation of the opposed edges of a surgical wound (Collins et al. 2002) as a result of inadequate strength during the early stages of healing or infection
- haemorrhage
- evisceration
- haematoma: clot formation between the opposed tissues that will impede healing.

To reduce the risk of postoperative complications the following steps may be taken:

- Patients should shower with shower gel/soap on the day of operation to remove dirt and transient skin bacteria.
- Patients should be provided with a clean theatre gown and clean bed sheets to reduce the likelihood of contamination with bacteria after they have showered.
- If necessary, hair should be removed from the operation site to allow access to the skin and prevent hair being trapped in the wound, preferably in theatre with clippers immediately before surgery.

Burns and scalds

Aetiology

Burns are traumatic wounds that may be caused by exposure to thermal extremes, caustic chemicals, electricity, radiation or direct heat (thermal). Severity is dictated by the strength of the causative factor and the duration of exposure or contact and is usually classified by the depth of the wound.

Every year over 100 000 people are treated in hospital for burns and scalds ranging from minor to fatal and a further 250 000 visit their GPs for treatment (Department of Trade and Industry or DTI 1999). Almost 45% of the injured are children under 5 years of age with 50% of these accidents happening in the kitchen. Almost 8000 people are admitted to hospital for treatment of burns and scalds and 211 people die each year as a result of their burn/scalding injury (DTI 1999).

The incidence of accidental burn and scald injuries is recognized as being higher in certain groups of people. Very young and elderly people are high-risk groups; men are more frequently affected than women in the 18- to 65-year age group (Dealey 2000). People who have epilepsy, obesity, neurological or cardiovascular disease with some degree of physical disability are more likely to suffer from burn and scalding injuries. People with stress, mental health problems and from lower socioeconomic classes are also more vulnerable. Non-accidental injury in children must be considered (Gordon and Goodwin 1997) and self-harm is commonly encountered in patients with mental health problems.

The effects of the injury should not be underestimated, from the initial pain and suffering to the long-term treatment, scarring and disfigurement, and psychological consequences, which can last for many years.

Types of burns

- Thermal burns: associated with misuse or mishandling of fire or combustible products such as matches or fireworks; they are the most commonly encountered burns. Exposure to extreme cold, steam or hot liquids and hot surfaces can also cause thermal burns.
- Chemical burns: direct skin contact with or inhalation of strong acids, alkalis or other corrosive substances; damage to vital organs may occur if chemicals are absorbed into the bloodstream (Dealey 2000).
- Electrical burns: caused by contact with high-voltage electrical current in the home, from outside transmission lines and lightning, flowing through the body. The extent of the damage internally may be more severe than is initially observed from the appearance of the skin wound and there may be associated thermal injury.
- Radiation: after radiation therapy or as a result of over-exposure to industrial ionizing radiation. Sunburn is the most common form after over-exposure to the sun.

Classification of burns and scalds

Burns are usually classified according to their depth. This can be from superficial, affecting the epidermis and upper section of the dermis, to a full-thickness burn involving the epidermis, dermis and subcutaneous tissue. Assessment will also involve estimating the percentage of total body surface area affected by the injury. The 'Rule of Nines' (for adults) and the Lund and Browder Classification (for children) are useful tools for obtaining relatively accurate estimates of the degree of damage.

Many burned patients are treated satisfactorily in local A&E departments; however, guidance is needed for those patients where the severity of the injury is such that specialist treatment in a burns unit is necessary.

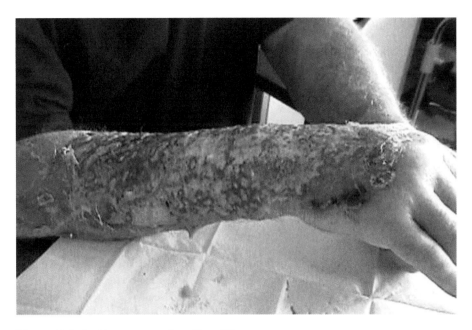

Figure 11.1 Scalds to an arm (see Plate 19).

The National Burn Care Review (2001) produced guidelines for transfer to a burns unit in the following circumstances:

- burns in patients under 5 years and over 60 years of age
- burns to the face, hands, feet or perineum
- any circumferential burns over joints
- inhalation injuries
- chemical and electrical injuries
- > 5% of the total body surface in a child
- > 10% of the total body surface in an adult
- any burn not healed in 14 days.

Treatment

As a first aid measure, the prompt application of cold water helps to stop the burning process and residual heat, and minimizes tissue damage (Lawrence 1981). Where the burn covers more than 10% of the body surface area, the application of water should be reduced to 5–10 minutes to prevent hypothermia (Edwards 2001). Initial assessment of the burn-injured patient should be carried out immediately after injury and should comprise assessment of the airway, breathing, circulation as a priority, level of consciousness and mobility:

- Airway: remove any obstruction.
- Breathing: observe chest movement on inspiration and expiration, its character and depth, to ensure that the patient is breathing normally.
- Circulation: check the pulse at the carotid artery and then the distal points to assess for shock or localized constriction.
- Level of consciousness: assess before attempting to move the patient.

Assessment of the severity, size and depth of the burn follows general patient support. In minor-to-moderate burns, the treatment comprises stopping the burning process and relieving pain. Smouldering clothing, bedclothes or other sources of heat should be removed and analgesics administered. The application of Clingfilm over the burn is advocated after the injury has cooled, to exclude air and bacteria, and to reduce excessive moisture loss and pain (Edwards 2001). The wound will be visible under the transparent covering which will be easy to remove without further trauma to the wound.

Once admitted to a health-care facility, the patient will undergo estimation of fluid loss and replacement by the intravenous route, if the loss is severe, to prevent hypovolaemic shock; vital signs will be monitored, pain will be controlled and further assessment of the injury made.

Pain may be more severe in superficial burn wounds than full-thickness wounds because the nerve endings are exposed. Suitable moisture-retentive dressings and regular analgesia should be provided.

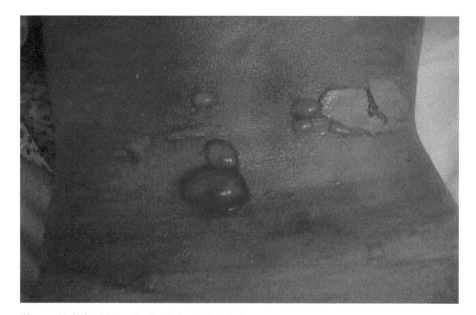

Figure 11.2 Scalds to the back (see Plate 20).

Special considerations

- Electrical burns: internal damage is usually greater than the external wound suggests; knowing the voltage involved may help the assessment. Life-threatening conditions such as ventricular fibrillation, cardiac or respiratory arrest may follow electrical burns.
- Chemical burns: irrigation with 0.9% saline or sterile water is recommended; the application of other solutions such as sodium bicarbonate may increase local heat, causing more tissue damage (Sciarra 2003). If the eyes are affected, they should be gently irrigated with sterile water or 0.9% saline for at least 30 minutes, then covered with a dry, sterile eye pad. The patient should be examined by an ophthalmologist.
- Location of the burn: possible loss of function must be considered when the burn injury affects the hands, feet, face or genitalia.
- Pre-existing medical conditions: conditions that affect the peripheral circulation may have a negative impact on healing, particularly diabetes mellitus, cardiovascular disease and substance abuse.
- Inhalation injuries: damage to lung tissue may exacerbate existing respiratory conditions.
- Age of the patient: those aged < 5 years and > 60 years are at higher risk of complications and therefore have a higher mortality rate (Sciarra 2003).
- Configuration of the burn: circumferential burns may lead to oedema which can impede blood flow to an extremity; neck or chest burns may obstruct respiration. Deep partial-thickness and full-thickness wounds cause permanent scarring and, after skin grafting or secondary intention healing, do not have the same characteristics as normal skin. The consequences may include restriction of joint mobility and cosmetic disfigurement.
- Psychological problems: a person who suffers burn injury may be physically and psychologically scarred for life. Post-traumatic distress syndrome, depression and diminished self-esteem caused by disfigurement may persist long after the injury has healed. A child's schooling and social activities may be severely curtailed while an adult may experience employment-related and relationship difficulties.

Dressings for burns

The range of treatments for burns varies enormously according to the depth, severity and extent of injury – there is no standard treatment (Edwards 2001). The management of the patient with major burns has been described; the local burn management is now outlined briefly.

Minor burns may be treated in the A&E or outpatient department but anyone with major burns must be admitted to hospital. The following people should be admitted for hospital treatment: those with > 5% of the total body area affected, burns on the hands, feet and genitalia, joints, face, history of electric shock, noxious vapour or inhalation, those with pre-existing medical conditions, e.g. epilepsy, small full-thickness burns, infection or septicaemia, suspected non-accidental injuries and elderly people (Gowar and Lawrence 1995).

The goals of burn management will be to:

- débride burn eschar if present
- promote rapid healing
- prevent/detect infection.

Surgical débridement, or the application of a dressing that will support autolysis (the body's own natural capacity for removing necrotic tissue as it uses its own enzymes to lyse, or break down, devitalized tissue – Collins et al. 2002), will assist removal of necrotic tissue. Silver sulfadiazine cream is the most widely used antibacterial treatment for burns to keep the bacterial count down before grafting. Silver sulfadiazine is effective against Gram-negative and Gram-positive pathogens, *Candida* sp. and yeasts. Aseptic dressing technique is vital at all stages of burn management.

Tulle and antiseptic-impregnated tulles have traditionally been used as easy to apply and cheap primary dressings for burns. However, they have been observed to adhere to the wound as they dry out, and granulation tissue grows into the open weave of the dressing causing trauma and pain on removal. Tulle dressings also cause maceration, shed fibres and restrict movement. In addition, personal hygiene will pose problems, because these dressings are not occlusive or waterproof and should not be allowed to become wet. Silver sulfadiazine cream is useful applied to the hands or feet and covered with a plastic bag to allow free movement of the fingers or toes. A drawback may be the accumulation of exudate in the bag with subsequent maceration; the bag will be heavy and may distort the wrist. Gore-Tex bags have been used more successfully because the fabric allows increased vapour permeability, preventing the accumulation of exudate in the bag (Terrill et al. 1991).

Hydrocolloids are suitable for low-to-medium exudate burn wounds because they have some degree of absorbency. Highly absorbent, flat foam dressings, sheet hydrogels, alginates, non-adherent wound contact layers and hydrofibre dressings will all be suitable for exuding burn wounds. The range of available dressings has now been complemented by the addition of silver-containing foam, hydrofibre, hydrocolloid and various wound contact layer dressings designed to reduce the bacterial count within the wound.

Dressing selection will follow the same guidance as for other wound types – assessment, clinical appearance, exudate levels, etc. – but the duration of use between dressing changes may vary until the exudate levels have stabilized after the first few days. Pain- and trauma-free removal is a prerequisite to good burn management and should be achieved through informed choice of products that will not adhere to the wound.

Patient information, in written form as well as given orally, should be provided about detecting early wound infection, i.e. the signs of inflammation, hand washing, the dressing, and how to care for the wound and use the dressing.

Cultured skin cells have been experimented with as treatments for burn wounds but the unit cost is high. However, they provide benefits in terms of quality of life, reduced healing time and hospital stay, and better cosmetic effect. This work is ongoing.

Scar care is important and patients should be given appropriate advice on how to minimize disfigurement. There is always the potential for hypertrophic scarring, which is red, raised and unsightly, and may cause contractures over joints. Non-perfumed emollients should be massaged into the healed scar to reduce this possibility. An alternative may be to apply a silicone gel sheet, which, in time, will flatten and soften the scar tissue. Protection of the scar tissue from the sun is essential for at least 12 months with a high factor sun cream.

Factitious wounds

Factitious wounds are those caused by self-wounding (Collins et al. 2002) and can be categorized as acute or chronic depending on the length of time present. Factitious disorders cover a wide range of psychiatric conditions in which patients portray themselves as ill. Little is known about who suffers from the condition, what causes it and how to treat it. The incidence of self-harm is sometimes difficult to identify, particularly in patients with immune system problems who present with wounds that do not heal with appropriate therapy or recur for no obvious reason. The patient may present with benign-appearing ulcerations that are not too painful and without systemic symptoms or infection, or deeper-seated infections in the joints where they may have been injecting noxious substances. The question that must be asked is: 'Does the patient do anything to perpetuate this disease process and wish to stay ill?' The typical appearance is that of a superficial wound located where the patient can reach it with the hand. This is not the place to go into the associated psychiatric problems but to say that self-harming patients will often have no shame, have an almost boastful attitude to their dilemma and relish the 'patient' role.

Attempting to develop a collaborative role with the patient combined with psychiatric assessment seems to be the key to recovery (Krahn 2003). Observation to confirm the diagnosis of factitious disorder and self-harm is desirable but not always possible. Good quality wound care with the appropriate medication, cognitive–behavioural therapy and psychotherapy as indicated by the psychiatric assessment will be required to aid healing. An example is shown in Figure 11.3.

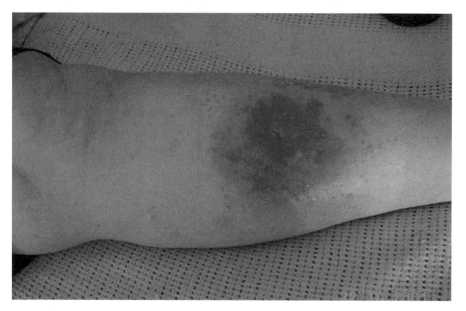

Figure 11.3 A factitious wound (see Plate 21).

Conclusion

This chapter has outlined the aetiology, diagnosis and treatment of a range of different acute wound types.

Student exercises

• Describe the first aid management of scalds.
• Name the factors that determine the likelihood of surgical wound infection.
• What signs would you look for in a patient you suspect of self-harming?

CHAPTER TWELVE

The incidence and prevalence of wounds

The epidemiology of wounds

This chapter provides limited epidemiological data and estimates of the size of the problem relating to pressure ulcers, leg ulcers, vascular wounds and diabetic ulcers. Information about the populations affected, age distribution and rates of recurrence (where possible) are presented. The difficulties encountered when attempting to obtain reliable epidemiological data are also discussed.

The primary purpose of any auditing process in health care is to improve patient care and clinical standards. Audit investigates present clinical practice and asks the question 'Is this best clinical practice?' It provides an important framework within which change can be implemented and monitored. The two main systems used for auditing pressure ulcers are incidence and prevalence, which can be used as an indication of improvements in standards of care (Collins et al. 2002). The former is used to gain a snapshot of all the patients in a defined population with pressure ulcers, and the latter to appraise the standard of care patients receive after contact with the health-care system. Whichever system is used for data collection the outcome should be change and/or improvement in practice; trends may be identified that were hitherto unknown, and measures taken to establish strategies for preventing tissue damage from an early stage.

Pressure ulcers

Pressure damage is common in all health-care settings and affects a wide range of patients. It is expensive both to prevent and to treat, it causes pain and suffering, and it is largely preventable.

A pressure ulcer is defined as an area of localized damage to the skin and underlying tissue caused by pressure, shear, friction and/or a combination of these (European Pressure Ulcer Advisory Panel or EPUAP 1999).

Elderly people are particularly susceptible with 70% of pressure ulcers occurring in patients over 70 years of age (Young and Dobrzanski 1992). There have been no UK-wide prevalence or incidence surveys conducted so the true extent of the problem is largely unknown.

Defining pressure damage in epidemiological and economic terms

Pressure ulcers are a largely avoidable complication of illness, disability or old age that affects the quality of life of patients in the whole range of care settings. Over time they have been known as pressure sores, decubitus ulcers and bed sores with the current term 'pressure ulcer' best describing their serious, disabling and sometimes fatal nature.

Hibbs (1988) suggested that 5% of pressure ulcers were inevitable despite preventive care and that 95% of established pressure ulcers could have been avoided. What is not known is whether preventive interventions would have had any impact on the development or otherwise of those that did occur. Patients entering health care with a medical condition should not expect to experience adverse complications often unrelated to their condition or treatment. Early identification of patients who are at risk of developing pressure damage is essential so that the appropriate interventions may be instigated as soon as possible.

Pressure ulcers rank as one of the four most expensive diseases to treat with cancer, cardiovascular diseases and AIDS (Haalboom 1991), and in the Netherlands account for 1% of the total costs of health care. Evaluating the financial burden of pressure ulcers is not sufficient; there must be a measure of health gain to balance the equation (Franks 2001). However, in the literature, there is much confusion about the number of individuals actually developing pressure ulcers. This confusion arises from different interpretations of the terms and different ways of measuring the occurrence of pressure ulcers: is the prevalence or incidence of pressure ulcers being measured? There are no clear epidemiological definitions so calculating the cost of both preventing and treating pressure ulcers is very difficult (Haalboom 2000).

The actual cost of both prevention and treatment to the NHS of pressure ulceration is known to be substantial (Cullum et al. 1995). In the UK the estimated cost of caring for patients with pressure ulcers is between £600 000 and £3 million a year (Touche Ross Report 1994) but there are several suggested variations in the figures proposed by other writers (Waterlow 1988, Department of Health or DoH 1991, 1993, McSweeney 1994), up to £300 million (Watkins 2000).

Following Hibbs's (1988) work, Collier (1999) calculated the cost of treatment of one patient with a grade 4 pressure ulcer to be £40 000. Treatment costs for patients with grades 0, 1, 2 and 3 were identified as

£2500, £7500 and £15 000–£20 000 respectively. These costs included staffing and extended hospital stay, whereas a similar Dutch study included 10% to cover the cost of special bed hire (Haalboom 1991).

The cost of prevention of pressure ulcers is the major drain on NHS resources in this area as a result of the large number of patients involved (DoH 1993) and because of extended length of hospital stay, the need for plastic surgery and greater dressing costs over time. Clark (1994) found the cost of treatment over 1 year in a district general hospital to be £78 228.93 compared with £90 118.35 for prevention as a result of the larger number of patients needing preventive care. Caring for people with severe pressure ulcers in the home has been found to have serious emotional, physical and financial impact on the lives of carers (Langemo et al. 2000).

Costs that are often overlooked are the opportunity costs associated with resources being used elsewhere which could be directed towards the care of others who may have their care delayed or even denied. In the modern NHS the focus is on reducing waiting lists, so a patient occupying a bed for longer than necessary would, in effect, be blocking the admission of one or more patients from the waiting list and using other resources.

Prevalence of pressure ulcers

There are two main methods for measuring the frequency with which pressure ulcers occur: prevalence and incidence. Prevalence can be defined as the number of people with a specific disease or condition as a proportion of a given population measured at a specific point in time (Dealey 2000). In hospitals, a point prevalence survey may be conducted over 1 day to identify the number of people with pressure ulcers. As a result of logistical difficulties in the community, it may be conducted over several days or 1 week to allow time for contact to be made with patients.

A prevalence survey provides useful information about the status quo, and the size and severity of the problem at the present time, but provides no evidence for why the pressure ulcers developed or whether patients are receiving a reasonable quality of care. Therefore, prevalence figures may be difficult to interpret and use in a meaningful way (Warner and Hall 1986).

The population or representative sample may be made up of hospitalized patients, the number of patients at risk, or the number of patients in the community or in a caseload, but they must be specified in advance. The prevalence rate constitutes a snapshot of all cases affected by the condition and so will include patients who have developed damage since admission to hospital or community care and those admitted with pressure ulcers. Some studies have been restricted to including specific groups of patients, e.g. children (Willcock et al. 2000), nursing home residents (Levett and Smith 2002) or general acute care hospital patients (O'Dea 1999).

The prevalence of pressure ulcers reported in UK hospitals ranges from 5% to 32.1%, in community settings from 4.4% to 6.8% and in nursing homes from 4.5 to 7.5% (Kaltenthaler et al. 2001). Fletcher (2001) reported that pressure ulcer prevalence ranged from 3% to 66% in the literature. A recent pan-European study of 5946 patients identified a prevalence of 18.1% (EPUAP 2002).

Prevalence surveys are time-consuming and labour intensive (auditors need training in risk assessment, grading of damage and data documentation), patients may be absent or missed for a number of reasons, with particular skills required for analysis, interpretation and reporting of the results. The recruitment and training of a number of data collectors to conduct the survey may lead to poor inter-rater reliability, because much of the assessment is subjective. The overall picture relates only to the time of monitoring and may change dramatically over hours or days, particularly in hospitals with new admissions and discharges.

Incidence of pressure ulcers

Incidence describes the continuing occurrence of new cases of a disease (Friedman 1994). Alderson (1983) defines the incidence rate as 'the number of patients developing a particular condition in a geographical area during a time period, divided by the estimated average population at risk'. Dealey (2000) believes that incidence surveying has the advantage that it is more sensitive than prevalence, providing more detailed and active data about the size and severity of the problem, and the quality of clinical practice. Improvement or deterioration of pressure damage may be tracked and monitored over time. Bridel-Nixon (1997a) believes that incidence is a useful measure of the extent of the burden created by short-lived or quickly recoverable diseases or problems. This means that a system must be established that is easy to operate, harnesses all the available data, and produces meaningful, accurate and usable results.

Hampton (1997) suggested four reasons for obtaining pressure ulcer incidence data:

1. to establish a baseline measure
2. to be able to assess performance in reducing pressure ulcer incidence
3. to determine educational requirements
4. to allocate resources efficiently.

The quality of care should be questioned if a patient develops pressure damage after entering into health care. However, it is not always possible to pinpoint exactly when a pressure ulcer developed because sometimes this will happen over a number of days before there are visible external signs. So hospital-acquired pressure ulcers may be starting before the patient is actually admitted but not be evident until after admission.

There is a degree of control over the potential for pressure ulcer development in newly admitted patients, which is measurable through accurate incidence monitoring. The correct clinical interventions applied at the right time are said to prevent most pressure ulcers occurring (Waterlow 1985, Hibbs 1988).

The reporting of pressure ulcer incidence studies is quite rare in the literature (Clark and Watts 1994) possibly as a result of the complexity of data collection. Some studies have concentrated on specific care groups, e.g. palliative care (Galvin 2002), critical care (Phillips 2000), lower limb amputees (Spittle et al. 2001) and other larger varied populations (Williams et al. 2001). From the published studies pressure ulcer incidence is seen to vary widely between 1.7% and 37.7% but how reliable the data collection methods, methodology or method of analysis has been is not known. Weaknesses in reported data mainly relate to:

- reliance on the motivation of staff to submit data
- inaccurate grading of the ulcers as a result of lack of skills and knowledge
- unreliability of assessment tools or unfamiliarity with assessment methods
- seasonal variations
- operational difficulties
- pressures of work.

In most cases, data are collected retrospectively, manually, using paper-based or computerized systems, which are both open to misuse and have a tendency to produce incomplete data. Pressure of work is a significant issue as the volume of paperwork that nurses are asked to complete escalates. Paperwork is generally not viewed as a priority when patients need attention. Another issue relates to who should complete assessments and incidence reporting forms: should this always be a first level nurse or is it acceptable for a health-care assistant to assess? The National Institute for Clinical Excellence (NICE) guidelines (2001) state that 'risk assessment should be carried out by personnel who have had appropriate and adequate training to recognise the risk factors that contribute to the development of pressure ulcers and how to initiate and maintain correct and suitable preventive methods'.

The aim of prevention and how to achieve success

Several authors have expressed concerns about lack of or poor knowledge about pressure ulcers within the nursing profession (Anthony 1987,

Alterescu and Alterescu 1992, Flanagan 1993, Xakellis 1993). The quality of the data collected must, therefore, be viewed with a degree of suspicion in terms of its completeness and accuracy. The use to which it is put should be carefully considered because purchasing decisions and training plans may be developed based on inadequate information. As for comparing total organizational progress with regard to pressure ulcer prevention, a reduction in the incidence rate may be linked to under-reporting, unreliable reporting or no reporting at all.

The activities of pressure ulcer monitoring provide methods for measuring, monitoring and establishing where there are flaws in the current patient management system. Both systems yield important data but decisions need to be made, based on local knowledge, expertise, IT systems and resources, on which is most relevant to local need. The processes involved in setting up both systems of monitoring are complex, but are valuable ways of appraising the quality of care and making nurses think about what they are doing and how care can be improved.

Leg ulceration

Epidemiology

Leg ulceration is a commonly encountered problem mainly found in elderly women. Leg ulcers are distributed fairly equally in both sexes up to the age of 40 years with the ratio increasing noticeably in women after the age of 65 years. Over 85 years of age the ratio of venous leg ulceration increases to 1:10.3 male:female; this is attributed to the fact that women live longer than men and to the increased risk of deep vein thrombosis during pregnancy in women (Callam et al. 1985). There are the psychological costs to the patient as well as the monetary costs to the NHS, as it is now well recognized that leg ulceration causes pain, affects sleep, restricts mobility and adversely affects self-esteem, possibly resulting in depression (Franks et al. 1994, Hamer and Roe 1994, Hyland et al. 1994, Anderson 1995, Price and Harding 1996).

Defining leg ulceration

Leg ulceration is defined as 'a loss of skin below the knee on the leg or foot which takes more than six weeks to heal' (Dale et al. 1983). The most common underlying cause of leg ulceration is chronic venous insufficiency/hypertension (70–75%), often mixed with arterial disease (10–20%). Other causes include peripheral vascular disease (10–15%), rheumatoid arthritis (10%), neuropathic (associated with diabetes mellitus) (5%), infection, trauma and inflammatory disease (Nelson 1995).

With a prevalence of between 1% and 2% of the UK population (Laing 1992), leg ulceration constitutes a major drain on health-care resources. This figure translates to between 80 000 and 100 000 patients with an active ulcer at a given time. Point prevalence surveys of leg ulceration conducted in the UK have revealed rates of between 1.5/1000 and 1.8/1000 people (Callam et al. 1985). Approximately 1.5–3.0 of the population has active venous leg ulcers at a given time (Cornwall et al. 1986). Gilchrist (1989) estimated that the number of people receiving treatment for leg ulcers is about 400 000. With approximately 400 000 people with a healed leg ulcer that is likely to recur (Callam et al. 1985), the costs of treatment are expected to continue to rise nationally.

Costs associated with treating patients with leg ulceration

The estimated cost of treating patients with leg ulcers is between £300 and £600 million p.a. (Collier 1996), which equates to 2% of the total health-care budget, and recurrence levels are high. The most expensive and significant resource used to treat leg ulcers is that of nursing time to assess and treat leg ulcer patients in the community (Nicholls 1990, Bosanquet 1992, Nelson 1995). One study reported that over 13% of all district nurse visits were treating leg ulcers (Value For Money Unit 1992). Community nurses have the disadvantage of working largely alone with little peer support, which can lead to isolation without the opportunity to share knowledge, experience and best practice with their peers. A study by Lees and Lambert (1992) showed that 70% of ulcers were being dressed more than once a week.

Over the last 10 years, there has been an upsurge in the volume of education offered to nurses about leg ulcer management, based on the encouraging results from various clinical studies and government initiatives (Royal College of Nursing or RCN 1998). Many UK community/primary care trusts have established leg ulcer services where compression bandaging is the gold standard for treating venous ulcers and fast-tracking systems are in place to expedite the treatment of patients with arterial and neuropathic leg and foot problems. Large numbers of district nurses have developed specialist skills through attendance at leg ulcer courses and study days. As a result, ulcers that may have been open for many years have been healed (Moffatt et al. 1992).

In spite of this, appropriate care may be disrupted if a patient is admitted to hospital, because little attention has been paid to providing hospital nurses with the appropriate knowledge and skills in leg ulcer care (Dealey

1999). There have not been any up-to-date prevalence surveys, but the RCN Sentinel Audit is hoping to persuade NICE to develop further the work from the audit pilot sites to cover the UK. The audit results will provide a good insight into current practice and whether it is evidence based.

Ischaemic or vascular wounds

Chronic lower limb ulceration caused by vascular aetiology presents the clinician with many complex and varied management problems. For the patient, pain, reduced mobility and impaired quality of life are major considerations. The primary aim of treatment is limb salvage with secondary aims of re-vascularization and prevention of infection in the compromised limb. A multidisciplinary approach to patient management that involves the patient in decisions about his or her care is the key to success.

Peripheral vascular disease is a progressive, inflammatory form of atherosclerosis where fatty degenerative plaques of fat are deposited on the inside walls of the larger arteries and harden (hardening of the arteries). The process continues until the artery walls are no longer elastic and have narrowed considerably. Therefore, peripheral vascular disease is a problem with narrowing of the lumen of the arteries in the limbs, which results in poor oxygen delivery to the areas beyond the narrowing. Cells require a baseline level of oxygen for survival. When this level is reduced, the local tissue dies and, with it, the capacity to regenerate. Thrombosis and total occlusion may occur as a result of advanced disease.

This condition is most likely to occur in the peripheral vessels such as the iliac, femoral and popliteal arteries supplying the legs, the renal arteries supplying the kidneys, the carotid arteries supplying the brain and the subclavian arteries supplying the arms. The arterial changes are exacerbated by hypertension and precede age-related degeneration of the body organs.

Prevalence of peripheral arterial disease

Peripheral arterial disease is commonly found in male smokers over the age of 50 years. The male:female ratio is 2:1 between the ages of 50 and 70 years (Dormandy and Ray 1996, Kumar and Clark 2001). Intermittent claudication (leg pain and weakness brought on by exercise and relieved by rest in a patient with arterial disease – Collins et al. 2002) is present in 5% of the population between the ages of 55 and 75 years and 10% of affected patients have diabetes. Approximately 50 000 people are hospitalized for the treatment of peripheral artery disease each year (Fowkes et al. 1991), consuming a large proportion of the health-care budget.

For further details of the prevalence of peripheral arterial disease, arterial ulcers and the risk factors for developing them see Chapter 10 (pages 115–151).

Outcome of care

Limb preservation is the goal of management by avoiding sepsis, further deterioration of the ulcer and vascular supply and, ultimately, amputation of the limb. One of the greatest difficulties associated with the care of patients with vascular disease is persuading them to change their lifestyle, in particular achieving smoking cessation. These sentiments are summarized by Goodall (2001), who states that medical management and advice are frequently thwarted or complicated by patients not complying with recommended regimens.

All surgical procedures carry risks that must be explained to the patient; treatment choices have to be balanced against what will happen if, for example, surgery is not carried out.

The underlying cause of any wound must be identified before attempts at management are made, not least in the case of vascular wounds. Here, there is the possibility of severe irreversible damage, possibly leading to amputation if the treatment is inappropriate. There is irrefutable evidence that smoking is one of a few correctable, direct causes of peripheral vascular disease but also one of the most difficult to influence in patients with the condition. Globally, emphasis on prevention of peripheral artery disease is vital, with much of the responsibility for disease prevention and prevention of complications being placed in the patient's hands. This is not so easy to achieve which is why so many more men and women are suffering the effects of peripheral artery disease.

Diabetic foot ulcers

Epidemiology

The World Health Organization predicts that the number of people with diabetes in developing countries could more than double in 30 years, from 115 million to 284 million (WHO 2003). Type 2 (non-insulin-dependent) diabetes mellitus accounts for about 90% of the total affected population, but the incidence of type 1 (insulin-dependent) diabetes mellitus is increasing in all age groups, mainly in the under 5 years, and of type 2 across all age groups and people from black and minority ethnic groups. Type 2 diabetes occurs when the body produces insulin either ineffectually or in inadequate amounts. Most people with type 2 diabetes also have some degree of insulin resistance, where the cells in the body are not able to respond to the insulin that is produced. More Europeans are susceptible to developing the disease partly because the average body weight has increased, so that in many cases the body is no longer able to maintain normal blood glucose levels (Lipsett 2003).

The implications of these increases will mean that a population of 100 000 would be expected to include between 2000 and 3000 people with diabetes, of whom approximately 25–30 will be children. These numbers will be significantly higher in those parts of the country with higher proportions of people from black and minority ethnic groups. Significant inequalities exist in the risk of developing diabetes, in access to health services and the quality of those services, and in health outcomes, particularly with regard to type 2 diabetes. Those who are overweight or obese, physically inactive or have a family history of diabetes are at increased risk of developing diabetes. People of south Asian, African, African–Caribbean and Middle Eastern descent have a higher than average risk of type 2 diabetes, as do less affluent people. Socially excluded communities, including prisoners, refugees and asylum seekers, and people with learning disabilities or mental health problems may receive poorer quality care. An estimated 500 000 UK Asians have diabetes and are six times more likely than white people to develop diabetes; up to 25% of UK Asians have diabetes compared with 5% of white people (John 2003).

Costs associated with treatment of patients with diabetic foot ulcers

The acknowledgement by the Department of Health (DoH 2001a) that diabetes is a life-long disease which can have a profound impact on lifestyle, relationships, work, income, health, well-being and life expectancy was reflected in the National Service Framework for Diabetes published in 2001. Diabetes impacts on the physical, psychological and material well-being of individuals and their families in many ways. Life expectancy is reduced as a result of higher mortality rates from coronary heart disease and stroke. Blindness, renal failure and risks associated with pregnancy are significant factors.

Costs associated with type 2 diabetes include direct and indirect personal costs of managing the diabetes. The average cost in 1999 was estimated to be £802 p.a. plus lost earnings. The development of diabetic complications increases personal expenditure threefold, and doubles the chance of having a carer (DoH 2001a). Costs to the NHS and Social Services are also significant with around 5% of total NHS resources (£23 million – Boulton 1994) and up to 10% of hospital inpatient resources currently being used for the care of people with diabetes because they are more likely to be admitted to and spend more time in hospital. The inpatient treatment of diabetic complications is high, as is the ongoing residential and nursing home care.

For further information on defining diabetic foot ulcers, peripheral neuropathy, peripheral vascular disease and their prevention, please see Chapter 10 (pages 115–151).

Student exercise

• Why are epidemiological data important?

CHAPTER THIRTEEN

Case studies

Case studies are an excellent way to learn about the detailed management of patients with different conditions, diseases or wounds. This chapter describes the nursing care of five patients who had complex wounds with complex underlying pathologies. Although most of the principles of wound care outlined in this book are adhered to, there are always exceptions to any rule. Each patient was referred for specialist advice because of the complexity of his or her illness and the way it was influencing the wound. The patient management and wound management are described because the two must never be considered in isolation – a holistic approach is vital to quality care.

The care of a patient with a pressure ulcer

This case study discusses the care of Olga, a patient admitted with a grade 3 pressure ulcer. The pressure ulcer occurred when Olga had been found in the bath at home 3 days after an epileptic seizure. The aetiology of the development of pressure ulcers is explained to aid understanding of the basic anatomical and pathophysiological changes involved and what can be done to prevent pressure damage.

Pressure ulcers

A pressure ulcer is defined as an area of localized damage to the skin and underlying tissue caused by pressure, shear, friction and/or a combination of these (European Pressure Ulcer Advisory Panel or EPUAP 1999). Pressure ulcers may present as one of the following:

- Grade 1: non-blanchable erythema of intact skin. Discoloration of the skin, warmth, oedema, induration or hardness may also be used as indicators, particularly on individuals with dark skin.

- Grade 2: partial-thickness skin loss involving epidermis, dermis or both. The ulcer is superficial and presents clinically as an abrasion or blister.
- Grade 3: full-thickness skin loss involving damage to or necrosis of subcutaneous tissue that may extend down to, but not through, underlying fascia.
- Grade 4: extensive destruction, tissue necrosis, or damage to muscle, bone or supporting structures with or without full-thickness skin loss.

A cascade of mechanisms occurs when the tissues are subjected to external damage from pressure, shear, friction or a combination of these factors, causing arterial, arteriolar and capillary vessel occlusion. This results in local anoxia, a sudden increase in blood flow (reactive hyperaemia) and the build-up of waste products. If pressure is of short duration, the result will be a return to normal in the tissues. If the pressure is not relieved, however, tissue necrosis will occur in the tissues situated between the skin and the bone (type 1 pressure ulcer – Barton and Barton 1981). The microcirculation is disrupted activating intrinsic clotting mechanisms and causing occlusion and ischaemic necrosis of the local tissues. Vital nutrients and oxygen cannot be delivered to the cells for metabolism so they die. Pressure damage can start to develop within 30 minutes in a vulnerable person. The only external sign of deep tissue damage may be discoloration of the skin, until a few days later when the extent of the pressure damage is revealed as the necrotic tissue sloughs off. A full-thickness ulcer will remain.

The patient – Olga

Olga was a pleasant, 67-year-old woman, of Polish origin, who lived alone. She spoke very little English, in spite of having lived in England for 30 years, but was able to understand simple questions and answer by nodding or shaking her head. On admission, she was alert but unable to provide any information about the cause of her injury or her medical history; nor was she registered at the trust. A neighbour had called the police when she had not seen Olga for 3 days and became concerned. With the assistance of an interpreter, a vague story emerged about how Olga had 'passed out' while taking a bath 3 days previously; she let the water out but could not get out of the bath or attract any attention to help her. Olga did not socialize but did have a daughter, who lived in London and visited her mother only infrequently.

Considering that Olga had spent 3 days in an empty bath, she was in fairly good general physical condition but unclear about why she was in hospital. An intravenous infusion was commenced to correct her dehydration and she was started on a soft diet as she had bitten her lip during the seizure.

It transpired that Olga had mild epilepsy treated by the GP but she rarely suffered from seizures.

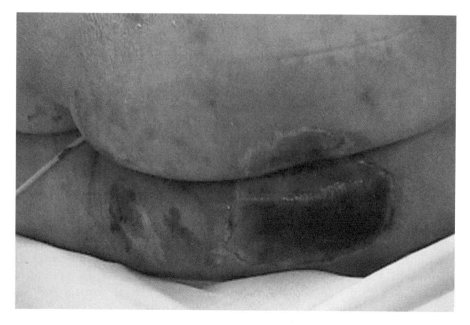

Figure 13.1 Sacral ulcer on admission (see Plate 22).

Assessment

On physical examination, Olga was found to have pressure damage to her sacrum and heels, the areas that had been in contact with the bath for 3 days. Non-blanching erythema of both heels suggested grade 1 pressure damage. Her sacrum was extensively discoloured with intact skin. A Waterlow assessment revealed a score of 15, high risk, as a result of immobility, recent poor nutritional intake and dehydration, damaged skin, mild obesity, female gender and her age. An alternating pressure air mattress (APAM) replacement was provided in anticipation of further tissue breakdown.

The pressure damage had occurred as a result of sitting on the hard surface of the bath for 3 days. During this time, the tissues had been subjected to very high pressures from her body weight for a long period, as she was unable to change her position. Shear forces are initiated when the skin remains in contact with the support surface (the bath) and a part of the body tries to move forward (the sacrum, heels); this would be happening as Olga tired and started to slide down in the bath.

Olga was confined to bed until the full extent of the sacral ulcer was realized, which took about 3 days. By this time, the discoloration had transformed into two deep cavities full of malodorous, necrotic tissue. As the days passed and the necrotic tissue separated from the viable tissue two large, deep, grade 3 pressure ulcers became visible.

Bed-rest was continued on the APAM with nutritional supplementation and local wound management. The grade 1 damage to the heels resolved within a few days; the sacral ulcers needed dressing daily to cope with large amounts of exudate and difficulty retaining dressings as Olga became more mobile in bed. The sacral ulcers were managed with hydrogel dressings covered with adhesive and foam dressings to aid de-sloughing, which were changed as required. Vacuum-assisted closure (VAC) therapy was applied when the wounds were clear of necrotic tissue and changed every 2 days until healing was complete. The Waterlow assessment was repeated every 2 days throughout her stay to ensure that nothing was changing to increase her risk of pressure damage. With Olga's permission photographs were taken every 2 weeks and tracings made to assess healing progress.

Use of the APAM continued until healing was complete with regular assisted re-positioning. Sitting was restricted until Olga's general condition allowed and it was safe, in view of the healing pressure ulcer, and then for only 1 hour at a time on a pressure-reducing cushion. Much time was spent trying to explain about the severity of the pressure damage and what was being done to aid healing. Olga's willingness to comply with treatment was a major contributory factor to successful healing.

The importance of the multidisciplinary team should not be underestimated: nurses including the tissue viability nurse, doctors, neurologist, therapists, social workers, dietitians and managers were involved in both the clinical and financial issues that arose from Olga's care.

Conclusion

Olga was lucky in that she was mobile and well nourished before the incident that caused her to be admitted to hospital. Although a stressful event, she appeared to recover psychologically quickly and was very patient while the ulcers were healing. The total healing time was 6 months, during which time she improved her English and obtained a home alarm system to avoid the possibility of such an event happening again.

The care of a patient with a leg ulcer

Leg ulceration is common, affecting 1–2% of the UK population (Laing 1982) and found mainly in very elderly people, particularly women, although 20% of leg ulcers are known to develop in the under-40 age group (Callam et al. 1985, Cornwall et al. 1986). Between 80 000 and 100 000 people have open ulcers and a further 400 000 have a healed ulcer that is likely to recur (Callam et al. 1985). Many leg ulcers persist over years as a result of an uncorrected underlying problem and in spite of appropriate management.

Leg ulcers are wounds of the lower limb, frequently chronic in nature, i.e. persisting for longer than 6 weeks (Cutting 1996). The causes of leg ulceration include chronic venous hypertension resulting from incompetent valves in the deep and perforating veins, arterial disease, and combined chronic venous hypertension and arterial disease (mixed ulcers). Other causes include neuropathy, vasculitis, malignancy, blood disorders, infection, metabolic disorders, lymphoedema, trauma, iatrogenic (ill-fitting plaster or bandage) and self-infliction (Morison and Moffat 1994).

Chronic venous insufficiency is the most common cause of leg ulceration and accounts for 70% of the total. Damage to valves in the veins of the leg arises from varicosities and thrombosis, and is responsible for later ulceration (Callam et al. 1985). Venous return is aided by the calf muscle pump, when it squeezes blood back up the legs into the general circulation against the force of gravity. When the valves are damaged, blood flows back towards the capillary bed, leading to venous hypertension and resulting in increased permeability of the veins that allow fibrinogen and red blood cells through into the tissues. The result is eczema, staining and thickening (fibrosis) of the tissues of the gaiter area of the leg (lipodermatosclerosis), which becomes fragile and easily damaged by minor trauma.

A number of theories have emerged that attempt to explain why venous ulcers occur, from the fibrin cuff theory (Burnand et al. 1982), white cell trapping theory (Coleridge-Smith et al. 1988), mechanical theory (Chant 1990), to the 'trap' growth factor theory (Higley et al. 1995).

Arterial disease, mainly atherosclerosis, accounts for about 10% of all leg ulcers. The effect of atherosclerosis reduces and/or blocks the arterial blood supply, typically to the lower leg, preventing the delivery of oxygen and nutrients to the cells. This can result in hypoxia and cell death, allowing minor injuries to result in skin breakdown and ulcer formation (Davis et al. 1992).

Other causes of leg ulcers include rheumatoid arthritis, diabetes mellitus resulting from small vessel vasculitis and disease, respectively, the presence of neuropathy and susceptibility to external damage from shoes, plasters, prostheses and bandages.

The patient – Sally

Sally was a 79-year-old woman living alone in a cottage in the country. She was slightly overweight and enjoyed a healthy diet, had reduced mobility as a result of osteoarthritis and rarely went out of the house. Carers visited daily to help with domestic chores and prepare Sally's meals, as she had no family living near by and few friends. She was taking non-steroidal anti-inflammatory medication for the osteoarthritis.

Sally had sustained a traumatic wound above her lateral malleolus 3 years previously that broke down and ulcerated, and which she initially self-treated. Her GP noticed the bandage some time later on a routine visit and asked the district nurse to assess and treat the wound. Doppler assessment showed an ankle–brachial pressure index of 0.9, indicating that the ulcer was the result of venous disease. Wound assessment revealed a sloughy, superficial ulcer measuring approximately 10 cm × 10 cm with moderate exudate. There was brown staining (haemosiderin) and ankle flare present with some eczema around the wound.

Treatment comprised multilayer bandaging to provide external gradu-ated compression from the base of the toes to below the knee. The aim was to support the superficial veins and counteract raised capillary pressure, to reduce oedema and promote healing. The implications of the proposed treatment with a four-layer compression bandage were discussed at length with Sally to ensure that she understood the importance of keeping the bandage in place. The skin of both legs was moisturized with 50% white soft paraffin/50% liquid paraffin to help to remove dead skin scales and debris after soaking for 5–10 minutes in warm water. A non-adherent dress-ing was applied before application of the bandage system, which consisted of a layer of padding, a layer of crepe bandage to smooth the first layer, a class 3a bandage (applied in a figure of eight) and a cohesive bandage.

Multilayer compression bandaging is bulky and warm to wear, so it is important to gain the trust and confidence of the patient before it is applied. Sally was advised to elevate her leg while sitting (above the level of the heart if possible) and to exercise the foot and ankle and walk to keep the calf muscle pump working, within her limit. Advice about finding footwear that would fit over the bandage helped compliance. Pain was a significant problem, so analgesia was prescribed and taken.

Sally managed the treatment well; the bandage was changed weekly when her legs were washed and moisturized, her pain level assessed, and the wound reassessed. Healing progressed until after 4 months the wound had healed. As a precaution against recurrence, Sally was prescribed compres-sion hosiery, which the carers helped her to apply, and the district nurse continued to visit monthly to check that there were no further problems.

Conclusion

This case study has described the relatively straightforward management of a compliant patient with a leg ulcer that healed with the correct treatment for her venous ulcer.

The care of a patient with an abdominal fistula

A gastrointestinal fistula can be defined as an abnormal communication between a part of the gastrointestinal tract and the skin or vagina (external) or between two parts of the gastrointestinal tract (Rinseina 1990) or, more simply, a track connecting two epithelial surfaces (Everett 1985). Fistulae can be a result of acquired or congenital conditions. Ileostomies and colostomies are surgically created fistulae but fistulae may arise spontaneously because of disease or after surgery. Other causes of external fistulae may be infection, obstruction, trauma or Crohn's disease (Borwell 1994). Everett (1985) states that the most common unexpected and unintended cause of fistulae is surgery usually as a result of the breakdown of an anastomosis, inadvertent damage to an organ or a loop of bowel becoming trapped between deep tension sutures. Examination of the discharge from the fistula will indicate which site it is connecting to, i.e. small bowel or large bowel. Fistula effluent may take the form of watery gastric juice, bile-stained fluid, faeces, urine or gastric contents.

Borwell (1994) suggests there are three different approaches to fistula management:

1. primary conservative treatment
2. immediate surgical treatment
3. no specific treatment because of patient-related or fistula-related factors.

The most frequently selected is the conservative approach with good patient support and preparation for surgery later. There are four key issues involved in patient management:

1. preservation of skin integrity
2. nutritional support
3. removal of odour and application of an effective, appropriate device
4. good communication of patient, carers and staff.

The patient – Tom

Tom was a 68-year-old retired agricultural engineer, living at home with his wife. One daughter was living locally and the older daughter 60 miles away. He had previously been a fit man and was a non-smoker but for the previous 4 years had been suffering from chronic hypoplastic myelodysplasia, thought to be associated with long-term anti-epileptic drug therapy. This condition equated to bone marrow failure which his sister also had. The chronic anaemia necessitated regular monthly blood transfusions, and later fortnightly, administered as an outpatient as his condition

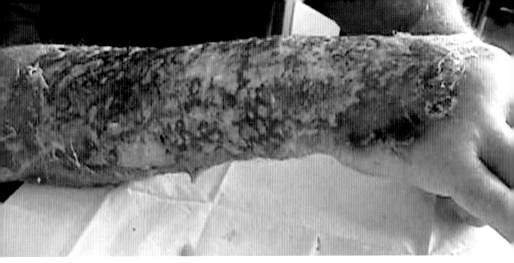

Plate 19 Scalds to arm.

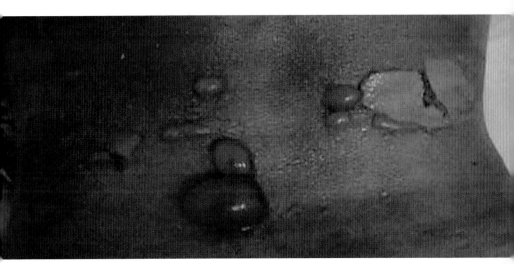

Plate 20 Scalds to the back.

Plate 21 Factitious wound.

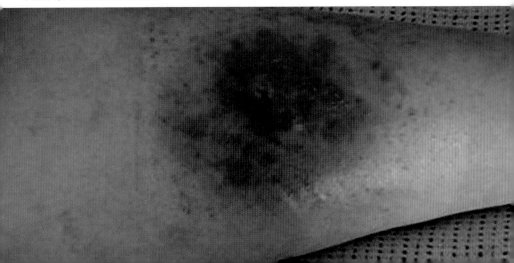

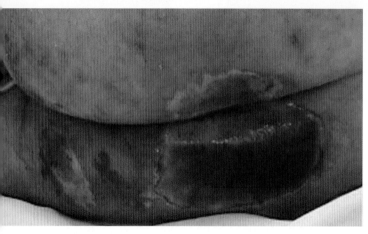

Plate 22 Olga – sacral pressure ulceration.

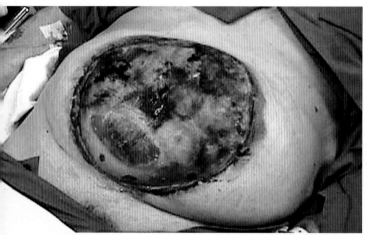

Plate 23 Abdominal fistula.

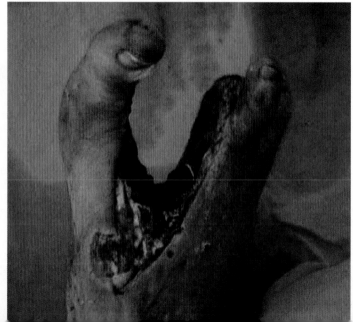

Plate 24 Ray amputation.

deteriorated. Tom's regular medication included carbamazepine for his seizures and atenolol for cerebrovascular disease. He had suffered a series of transient ischaemic attacks in the past and was allergic to penicillin.

Medical history

In May 2000 Tom underwent surgery for right iliac fossa pain. A gangrenous appendix was found and removed. A few days later, paralytic ileus developed, requiring a further laparotomy to release abdominal adhesions. Several serious complications ensued: septic shock, septicaemia, renal failure, jaundice and superficial dehiscence of the abdominal wound. The appendicectomy wound healed without complication. A month later, he was discharged to the care of the district nurses and his wound was checked regularly in the medical day unit when he visited for top-up blood transfusions. The laparotomy wound remained unhealed and persisted in this state until his admission to hospital 18 months later.

The wound before admission

There were two wounds: the upper wound, the smaller of the two, measured 7 cm × 7 cm, was circular and appeared to be granulating. The lower, much larger wound (15 cm × 15 cm) extended from the midabdomen to just below the umbilicus. The wound edges were ill-defined, dark and suggestive of a non-healing wound. There appeared to be dusky-coloured, fleshy, wet, granulation tissue over the main part of the wound with an area of capillary bleeding towards the lower edge. The umbilicus had been shifted about 13 cm to the left of his abdomen by the lower wound. A silicone, non-adherent dressing was being used to treat the upper half and an alginate one to try to stem the bleeding in the lower half of the wound. The whole wound was then covered with an absorbent, adhesive-bordered foam dressing which needed changing two to three times a day.

Hospitalization

Tom's general condition deteriorated, the wound became sloughy and malodorous and the bleeding increased (particularly after he had been transfused, his wife reported). Tom was admitted to hospital after collapsing at home. At this time his blood results gave real cause for concern with the haemoglobin at 6.9 g/dl (normal male 130–180 g/dl), white cell count $1.1 \times 10^9/l$ (normal $4–11 \times 10^9/l$) and the platelet count $10 \times 10^9/l$ (normal $150–400 \times 10^9/l$). Four units of blood were transfused immediately. The wound had extended to the point where both lesions had merged into one large wound of approximately 21 cm × 21 cm. The tissues looked very

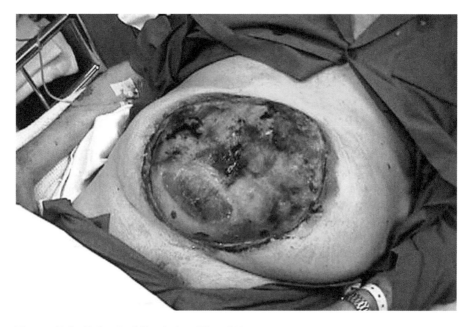

Figure 13.2 Abdominal fistula (see Plate 23).

fragile overall with no indication of healing at the wound edges. As Tom's condition worsened it was decided that surgical intervention would not be appropriate considering his poor condition, chronic anaemia, wound infection, the fragility of the tissues and the assumption that postoperative healing would be difficult to achieve.

Tom was pyrexial and wound swabs from the abdomen cultured *Staphylococcus aureus* for which the appropriate antibiotics, teicoplanin and ciprafloxin, were prescribed and administered intravenously. By this time his wife and daughter, who had been coping very well at home with Tom, were exhausted.

Five days later, the upper part of the wound remained static with no positive signs of healing. The appearance of the lower part of the wound started to change. The lower area of fragile tissue was extending in size and the exudate was changing. Three weeks later the abdomen was distended, the wound was larger and covered with dry necrotic tissue. The silicone dressing was continued to re-hydrate the wound and covered with adhesive, foam, absorbent dressings for occlusion and absorbency. Peristalsis could be observed across the lower part of the wound beneath the peritoneum.

A Hickman line was inserted specifically for blood transfusion but, on the failure of elemental feeding, had to be used for the administration of total parenteral nutrition (TPN). The dietitian was closely monitoring

Tom's progress and prescribing appropriate replacement diets to cope with the loss of protein, vitamins and other elements, plus the increased requirement for carbohydrate associated with trying to heal such a large wound.

Over the next 2 days the abdominal distension reduced so that the wound looked smaller but from seeping frank blood this changed to an excessive volume of what appeared to be semi-solid faecal matter that became bile stained after a few days. The wound was being re-dressed three to four times daily as before but, in spite of the frequency of dressing changes, the leakage was uncontrollable. There was a fistula connecting the small bowel with the wound, with the bleeding coming from the capillaries of the peritoneum.

Major problems arose concerning the skin surrounding the wound which was continually being subjected to the corrosive effects of gastrointestinal effluent. Within 24 hours there was evidence of severe skin damage. The area of affected skin around the wound was covered with a skin barrier film before dressings were applied and successfully helped to reverse the damage that had occurred.

At this point octreotide was administered by subcutaneous injection to reduce gastrointestinal secretions and therefore fistula effluent. Artificial saliva was used to keep his mouth moist and clean because Tom was not taking anything by mouth and he could not tolerate his teeth being brushed. An electric profiling bed and alternating pressure mattress were provided at an early stage because Tom was assessed as very high risk for pressure ulcer development and was difficult to re-position as a result of pain and weakness. Tom was becoming very depressed about his pain and his condition but was very well supported by his family. Fentanyl patches were administered finally with his wife's permission, on an increasing dose regimen to control his pain. Tom and his wife had both wanted him to stay alert for as long as possible. Gelifusin (a plasma expander) was transfused to correct fluid depletion on several occasions but his condition continued to deteriorate.

Wound management

When the fistula began discharging semi-solid faecal fluid, medical instructions were to set up a system of continuous low-pressure suction. This was done using a double thickness of film dressing with a catheter in contact with the site of the discharge connected to a drainage bag. This failed as a result of the size and shape of the wound and difficulties making the area air and fluid tight. Vacutex absorbent dressing was tried under the absorbent, adherent foam dressings, but it could not cope with the very high volume of effluent. It was decided that a drainable wound management bag, large enough to cover the whole wound, would be more suitable.

On measuring the wound and checking the available sizes of wound drainage bags there were none large enough from NHS Logistics Authority (NHS Supplies) to cover the wound which was now 25 cm across. Contact with a local stoma care representative resulted in access to wound drainage bags that would almost fit over the large defect. The back of the bag consisted of a large sheet of hydrocolloid from which a template of the wound was used to cut the correct size – slightly larger than the lower part of the wound to prevent seepage (Borwell 1994). The bag had an opening porthole for access to the wound for re-dressing and a drainage channel for easy measuring and removal of effluent. An absorbent, adherent, foam dressing was applied to the upper part of the wound to cover the part that lay outside the bag.

The method used for application was to cleanse the abdominal area with saline, apply Cavilon to the surrounding skin, apply thin hydrocolloid to the whole of the wound margin, then carefully apply the drainage bag (after warming the hydrocolloid backing) so that it adhered to the hydro-colloid and foam dressing and was air- and water-tight. The volume of effluent could now be drained and measured, but by this time it was obvious that little could be done for Tom. His family were staying at the hospital day and night and were involved throughout in all nursing and medical decisions about his care. The main advantage of using such an appliance was that Tom's wound needed minimal interference and was considered successful as each bag remained in place for at least 5 days until Tom's death 2 weeks later.

Conclusion

This case study has described the complex problems facing nursing and medical staff during Tom's stay in hospital until his death. The difficulties associated with obtaining a suitable drainage bag large enough to cope with the size of wound and volume of drainage were a challenge as was his need for skilled nursing care throughout his stay. Emotional as well as prac-tical support for Tom and his family was another particular challenge, especially as they had successfully managed his care at home for so long.

The care of a patient with a neuropathic diabetic foot ulcer

Foot disease in patients with diabetes is a major, often preventable, prob-lem and, although people with diabetes constitute 2% of the population, they will undergo 50% of all major amputations of a lower limb (Edmonds et al. 1996). The key to successful management is a team approach which includes input from specialist doctors, nurses and podiatrists (Foster 1999). Early detection, fast-tracking and treatment at specialist foot clinics for people with diabetes and foot problems is essential and has been proved to reduce major amputations by 50% (Edmonds et al. 1986).

Minor wounds or infections in feet with a normal blood supply and sensation are recognized by the pain experienced by the individual, and, hence, can be treated early and heal at the normal rate without complication. Patients with diabetes, with insensate feet and vascular perfusion, can avoid many of the apparently minor traumas that often lead to major foot problems by having an awareness of how their feet may be damaged. Once damage has occurred a lack of awareness of the damage, potential problems and subsequent removal of the source of the injury are often delayed, leading to irreparable damage.

Faris (1982) classified the factors responsible for the development of foot problems as predisposing and precipitating factors (Table 13.1).

Table 13.1 Factors responsible for development of foot problems

Predisposing factors	Precipitating factors
Vascular disease – ischaemia	Physical injury
	Mechanical trauma
	Heat
Neuropathy – loss of perception of pain	Infection
Liability to infection	

Of these factors, loss of perception of pain and ischaemia are the two most significant ones in the development of foot lesions. Arteriosclerosis is probably the most important factor causing non-healing of wounds as a result of reduced blood supply, and they may cause ischaemic pain at rest. Ischaemia potentiates the spread of infection by abnormal cellular and humoral response to inflammation, and dysfunction of the autonomic nervous system.

Minor trauma such as a puncture wound caused by an ingrowing toenail will allow ingress of bacteria, resulting in local infection. Pressure caused by tight shoes may cause pressure necrosis and repeated mechanical trauma from walking can cause inflammation and necrosis. Reduced sensitivity to pain and temperature, e.g. from a hot water bottle, may cause damage.

Vascular disease and neuropathy cannot be reversed but their onset may be delayed by avoidance of precipitating factors. Patients must try to avoid tissue damage from physical trauma and it is the responsibility of the health-care professional to educate patients with diabetes about how to protect their feet.

A recent Audit Commission (2000) report highlights the many deficiencies of the service currently provided for patients with diabetes. The audit found that only four of nine hospitals had a structured, multidisciplinary education programme and two-thirds of patients said that they had received no formal education in the last year. Perhaps, more importantly, one in five patient case notes had no record of a foot examination and half of the patients had been referred late with serious foot ulcers.

Figure 13.3 shows the interaction between predisposing and precipitating factors in the development of diabetic foot lesions.

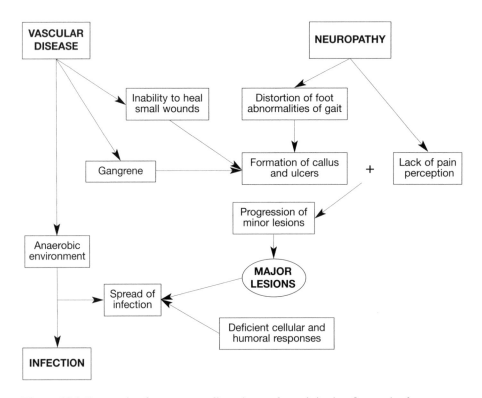

Figure 13.3 Interaction between predisposing and precipitating factors in the development of diabetic foot lesions.

The patient – Clive

This case study describes the care of a patient with diabetes mellitus who presented with a small, painless ulcer on the plantar surface of his right foot between the first and second metatarsal heads. The wound was treated surgically before being managed with a hydrofibre dressing. Management of the patient involved several members of the multidisciplinary team working together. The subject of this case study is Clive, an otherwise fit and healthy 62-year-old man, who runs a public house in a small village with his wife. The job requires long periods of standing in the kitchen, preparing food, and in the bar, serving customers. He and his wife had been on holiday in Tenerife before the development of the plantar ulcer, during which time they had spent a lot of time walking. Clive had been walking in sandals without socks. It is presumed that, as a result of his peripheral neuropathy, he was unaware of sustaining a minor penetrating injury to the sole of his foot and continued walking.

Clive had had type 2 diabetes mellitus since 1989. Since that time, his blood glucose levels had been well controlled with a sugar-free diet and oral medication. As a result of increasing and uncontrollable blood glucose levels, it became necessary to prescribe insulin 10 years later in 1999. Clive, a non-smoker, did admit to consuming about 8 units of alcohol daily. He had never attended a podiatrist for foot care and had been given no information about the importance of foot care or about the implications of peripheral neuropathy since his diagnosis of diabetes mellitus in 1989.

On admission to hospital, Clive's presenting problem was cellulitis of his right foot and leg with a painless, 'punched-out' ulcer under the right foot for the previous 4 days. Callus formation was evident on the weight-bearing surfaces of the foot. An infected neuropathic ulcer was diagnosed. Blood was taken for a full blood count, erythrocyte sedimentation rate, blood glucose and blood cultures, because he was pyrexial at 38°C on admission. Intravenous flucloxacillin, amoxicillin and metronidazole were administered, the foot was radiographed to exclude the presence of a foreign body or osteomyelitis, and Clive was referred to the hospital podiatrist. Doppler assessment revealed normal pulses.

Throughout his hospitalization, Clive was self-caring. The podiatrist attended the day after admission and documented a malodorous, necrotic, plantar ulcer, which she débrided with a scalpel. On examination there was evidence of further breakdown under the necrotic tissue. After débridement an absorbent foam dressing was applied and the patient advised not to weight-bear on the right foot. Prophylactic administration of heparin was prescribed during Clive's period of bed-rest to prevent deep vein thrombosis.

After 4 days of antibiotics, elevation and bed-rest the patient was reviewed. It was decided that, although the pyrexia was subsiding, the wound was unlikely to heal spontaneously. The erythema was spreading over the right great toe, foot and leg, which were becoming painful. The second toe was considered to be non-viable at this point. Local wound treatment with a hydrogel and absorbent foam dressing was making little difference. Referral was made for a surgical opinion that confirmed the view that the problem was more serious than was first anticipated. Clive was examined by the surgical consultant and transferred to a surgical ward. By this time it was evident that there was swelling and necrosis underlying the second metatarsophalangeal joint with proximal swelling of the plantar aspect; the second toe was not viable.

Surgery

Clive was warned of the seriousness of the problem and that the proposed ray amputation, if unsuccessful, may necessitate further lower limb amputation. Ray amputation (amputation of the right second toe – Figure 13.4) with extensive débridement of the plantar surface, excision of the metatarsal and wide débridement of necrotic tissue was performed the next day.

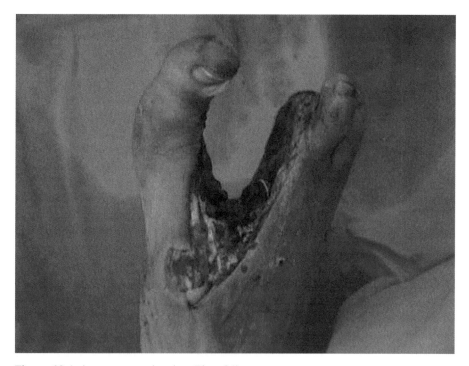

Figure 13.4 A ray amputation (see Plate 24).

Ray amputation

The aim of carrying out the ray amputation was to excise non-viable tissue but, more importantly, to preserve a useful foot. This is a local amputation which, if it is found that there is an insufficient vascular supply, may lead to a major amputation. There are certain 'rules of thumb' followed by surgeons when dealing with diabetic foot problems as follows:

• thorough but gentle exploration and excision
• tourniquets should not be used
• wide incisions to allow drainage are preferable to small incisions – healing will take the same length of time if the blood supply is adequate
• the other foot must be protected at all times (Faris 1982).

The ray amputation (Figure 13.4 and Plate 24) is considered to be the most useful because it provides excellent drainage from the deep parts of the foot. Once infected, there is always the danger of infection spreading through the foot.

The incision encircles the base of the toe extending proximally into the sole of the foot with disarticulation at the metatarsophalangeal joint. The bone is divided at the midshaft of the metatarsal. The technique allows wide drainage of blood and infected material from the deep tissues. Postoperative bandaging exposes the remaining toes for inspection and palpation. Great care and attention is necessary postoperatively both to ensure good healing and for early detection of signs that may indicate that further major amputation is required.

Postoperative recovery and wound management

Clive made an uneventful recovery from his operation. Following the perioperative Alberti regimen, his insulin was recommenced 24 hours after surgery and blood sugars remained stable. The wound had been packed with an alginate dressing that was removed and replaced after 24 hours. Wound assessment at this point revealed a very deep incision with a moderate amount of exudate. The dressing was changed to a hydrofibre dressing to absorb exudate, keep the wound free of further necrotic material and maintain optimum conditions for healing. As expected, there was evidence of necrosis and slough formation within the moist wound after 3 days, for which the hydrofibre dressing was appropriate.

Hydrofibre dressings are second-generation hydrocolloids that absorb up to 25 times their weight in fluid without losing the integrity of the dressing. They consist of carboxymethylcellulose, which gels on contact with fluid. The mode of action is different to conventional dressings in that hydrofibre dressings absorb fluid by hydrophilic action. Fluid is absorbed directly into the fibre structure, which is said to increase significantly the volume that can be retained within the dressing. An important advantage relates to the method of absorption, which is by vertical wicking rather than lateral wicking so keeping moisture locked in the dressing and away from surrounding skin. Hydrofibre dressings are available in sheet and rope presentations and on FP10.

During the 10 days postoperatively, and as there were no signs of clinical infection, the dressing was changed every 2 days. At each dressing change, the wound was cleaner and granulation tissue was evident after 1 week.

Joint management between the vascular nurse and podiatrist ensured that the foot was protected with adequate padding. Later, a plaster sandal padded with orthopaedic felt to relieve all pressure from the operated area of the forefoot was provided. The patient was taught to non-weight bear with crutches, advised to limit his mobility and to take plenty of rest with his leg elevated.

Discharge

Clive was discharged 10 days after surgery with a very deep wound that was expected to take several months to heal. During the healing period the build-up of dead skin, callus and necrotic tissue was gently removed by the podiatrist from the edges of the wound whenever necessary at clinic visits. Clive attended the clinic fortnightly for re-dressing and inspection with the district nurse changing the dressings every 2 days in between. The hydrofibre dressing was used throughout and provided comfortable and effective wound management. Advantages associated with this product included instant gelling to provide a moist environment and immediate exudate management.

Conclusion

This case report outlines the care of a patient with diabetes for a condition that could have been avoided if the right information had been given and acted upon. The Audit Commission (2000) states that patient education is at the heart of good diabetes care and self-management is the key to successful diabetes care. Many deficiencies relating to both clinical assessment of the feet of patients with diabetes and general diabetic patient education were found. Many complications can be avoided or at least deferred by appropriate self-care such as looking after the feet. Clive was taught how to inspect his feet, what to look for, what conditions to avoid, e.g. walking barefoot, and given an information leaflet explaining diabetic foot care.

Foot care advice

People with diabetes should be given verbal and written advice from their first contact with a health-care professional. This may be the practice nurse, diabetes nurse specialist, podiatrist, community or hospital nurse.

Diabetics' feet should be formally examined on initial contact and at least annually and they should be taught how to inspect their own feet regularly. Advice should include:

- wear shoes or slippers – never go barefoot
- do not use tight garters
- wear well-fitting shoes not tight or worn shoes; wear boots only for a short time
- wear socks inside out to avoid pressure from seams
- wash feet daily and check them for blisters, cuts and scratches
- keep feet dry especially between the toes; use unscented powder if needed
- do not let the skin get dry and cracked – use moisturizer
- do not use hot water, only lukewarm; no heating pads, hot water bottles, Epsom salts, iodine or alcohol should be used
- cut toenails straight across not deep into corners
- never use knives, razors or corn treatments
- feel inside your shoes for sharp objects
- if your vision is impaired get someone else to check your feet
- consult your podiatrist, doctor or nurse about foot problems immediately.

The care of a patient with a fungating malignant wound

Foul-smelling, fungating, malignant tumours present a major clinical challenge to the clinician (Grocott 1995b). Cleansing and management of these wounds is difficult, with exudate that is copious and offensive in areas that are in close proximity to the patient's nose and the presence of friable, bleeding tissue.

The patient – Jane

An elderly woman, Jane, was admitted to a general surgery ward with a foul-smelling fungating carcinoma of her left breast. She had been living with her older sister and they looked after each other. There was no recollection of when the problem with her breast had first appeared and she had not mentioned it to her GP until immediately before admission to hospital and therefore had not received treatment of any kind.

The malignant lesion extended from the sternum under her axilla through to her back, and, in depth, down to her rib cage. The wound was sloughy, bleeding and malodorous on assessment. The breast tissue had been completely destroyed, leaving a large cavity that extended from her chest through her axilla and around her back.

Jane was oriented and chatty and appeared to enjoy the attention she was being given. Initially she was able to walk to the toilet with help and sit out in a chair comfortably, and her appetite was good. In spite of the extent of the lesion, Jane never complained of pain; her main concern was that the nurses had to cope with the odour. In view of the extent of the lesion, no active medical or surgical treatment was proposed because she was considered to be terminally ill. Effective wound management, pain control and general nursing support, when needed, were going to be the priorities for Jane. The ward nurses contacted the tissue viability service for advice about how to manage the patient and her wound.

Patient assessment

Following patient and wound assessment the following were priorities for care:

* to try to stem the bleeding
* to clean the wound
* to control the odour
* to manage the excessive amounts of lymph fluid and exudate being produced
* to prevent infection
* to establish a dressing regimen that caused as little disturbance as possible to the patient
* to provide a dressing that was unobtrusive and comfortable.

Although the objectives were clear, actually to achieve them required a large degree of creativity as well as knowledge, skill and experience.

Dressing regimens

Following gentle irrigation with warmed saline the first dressing regimen consisted of five alginate ribbon dressings (with haemostatic properties) covered with odour-absorbing dressings that contained activated charcoal and silver, secured with absorbent, adhesive foam dressings. The surrounding skin was protected with a skin sealant reapplied every 3 days as a precaution, knowing that dressing changes would be frequent and expecting maceration from the excessive amounts of exudate. This combination lasted on average 8–12 hours before the fluid, aided by gravity, seeped through the bottom half of the foam dressings.

The second dressing regimen comprised hydrofibre dressings, odour-absorbing dressings, dispersion dressing and non-adhesive foam dressings secured with tape around the edges. Again, the problem was related to the fluid seeping downwards and not being absorbed throughout the whole of the absorbent dressings. This combination of dressings lasted about 12 hours.

In desperation, contact was made with several companies and experts to ask whether they had any suggestions. One expert suggested 'nappies', which seemed rather unorthodox, but looking at the shape of the absorbent insert used in incontinence pants it was ideal, i.e. wider at one end and tapering to a narrower part, and very absorbent. These were taped over the sealed secondary dressing to good effect; there was no leakage on to Jane's nightclothes. Another good idea proposed by a member of the team was to use stretch net pants placed over the body with the patient's arms through the leg holes and a hole cut in the gusset for the head. This proved to be an excellent way to retain the bulk of the dressing very neatly and was a source of great amusement to the patient and staff.

The whole range of absorbent foam dressings was worked through, each having claims that it was more absorbent and that it absorbed laterally as well as vertically, with little success. Finally, a dressing regimen that incorporated a product not yet available in the UK was adopted. The product is a sachet of highly absorbent hydrocolloid beads, which is placed in the wound to absorb exudate, debris and bacteria from the wound surface. The granules take up the exudate to form a gel on the wound contact layer. The features of this dressing incorporated absorbency, reduction of odour and cleansing of chronic wounds. Unfortunately the product is available only in small sized 'teabags', 5 cm × 5 cm, so several were needed to fill the wound. The regimen included foam absorbent dressings and, after a few days, the odour-absorbing dressing was omitted because the wound was much cleaner and much less foul smelling. This combination lasted between 12 and 24 hours and appeared to be meeting all the objectives that had been set. Metronidazole was not prescribed orally because of its unpleasant gastrointestinal effects, and was not necessary locally as the wound became cleaner and less malodorous.

The patient was happy that the wound no longer smelled, that her night-clothes were dry and that the nurses did not have to change the dressings so frequently. Jane was involved in management decisions as far as possible and took an active interest in the clinical deliberations about the pros and cons of different dressing choices.

It was impossible to calculate the total cost of the dressings used because many were generously supplied by the dressing companies. As an example, an approximate 24-hour cost of one of the early dressing regimens would have been in the region of £42. Jane died after 4 weeks in hospital, experiencing pain only for the last few days for which she had analgesia via a pump. The ward nurses were satisfied that they were providing the best management under very difficult circumstances.

Conclusion

A suitable dressing regimen was achieved after about 10 days of experimenting with the different dressing combinations. This was an unusually difficult wound to manage and the fact that so many different dressings were used did not detract from their effectiveness under less complicated conditions. Choices of products used in combination were based on existing knowledge and experience supplemented by that of colleagues in the field of tissue viability, company representatives and nurse advisers. Following wound assessment, the properties and characteristics of each product were carefully considered to allow informed, safe and clinically defensible choices to be made.

Overall conclusions

No two wounds are the same; nor can blanket treatment be applied in all cases. Every patient must be treated as an individual, with needs that are unique to him or her. The nurse must consider all the available options for care and decide which is most suitable, taking into consideration acceptability to the patient, evidence of effectiveness and, finally, cost.

Student exercises

- Discuss how you would manage a patient who refused multilayer compression bandaging.
- What advice would you give to a patient with diabetes and a wound?
- How would you help a patient with a fungating malignant wound psychologically?

CHAPTER FOURTEEN

Professional guidance for practitioners

Professional regulation and wound care practice

It is the duty of every health-care practitioner to be aware of and understand the contents of their codes of professional conduct as well as relevant legislation governing their practice. The NMC *Code of Professional Conduct* (2002b) states that as a registered nurse, midwife or health visitor you are personally accountable for your practice. In caring for your patients you must:

- respect the patient or client as an individual
- obtain consent before you give any treatment or care
- protect confidential information
- cooperate with others in the team
- maintain your professional knowledge and competence
- be trustworthy
- act to identify and minimize risk to patients and clients.

The implications for practice of each of these elements of the *Code of Professional Conduct* are discussed in relation to tissue viability.

Respect the patient or client as an individual

Health-care professionals must promote the interests of patients at all times. Patients, where possible, should be respected and fully involved in the decision-making process for their care. In the case of patients who are unable to participate in this process for physical or psychological reasons, relatives and carers should be provided with information and brought into the discussion. The approach to all patients must be consistent, irrespective of culture, age, gender, race, ability, sexuality, economic status, lifestyle, or religious or political beliefs. Important information relating to the patient's health state, previous wound treatments, allergies and preferences may be obtained and considered. Decisions to use different dressings or therapies must be talked through before their application, e.g. the application of maggots to a wound will be totally unacceptable to a small number of patients, whereas other patients, for whom various alternative therapies have failed, would welcome the opportunity. This is particularly the case in patients with diabetes who know that the alternative to attempts at healing is lower limb amputation. Details of any therapy, its risks and potential benefits must be explained in language that the patient understands and backed up with written information.

Obtain consent before you give any treatment or care

Following on from the explanation of a treatment or therapy to the patient should come their informed consent to the proposed treatment. Informed consent implies that the patient has heard and understood the explanation, and is in a position to make a decision and willing to proceed with the treatment. This is where the risks and benefits will have bearing on whether patients wish to take the chance of the treatment not living up to their expectations or failing. In the case of patients refusing to undergo a treatment, their wishes must be respected with no detriment to their future care.

Patient consent to participation in a clinical trial of new dressings, for example, may result in randomization into the standard treatment group. Informed consent is still required for participation and, usually, for photographs to be taken and used in the ways stated on the consent form and patient information sheet. Patients must be aware that images of their wounds may be subsequently seen by and used for analysis by companies sponsoring the research. Patients should never be identifiable from any photographs taken of them and/or their wounds. Patients have the right to refuse to participate in a trial and under any circumstances can refuse to have photographs taken without their consent.

Protect confidential information

All information collected about patient care should be treated as confidential. Obviously, members of the multidisciplinary team caring for the patient must have access to ensure that patient care is not compromised by ignorance of a significant event or incident. Rules vary between organizations regarding the location of nursing, medical and therapy documentation; it may be found at the bedside or at the nurses' station. There may be white boards, on which patients' names are written, strategically located on wards and in departments where health-care practitioners, patients, visitors and others can read them. These are locally agreed decisions that must consider the possibility of breach of confidentiality.

Again, clinical trial data are confidential and should be held in safe physical storage or, if stored on computer, be password protected, the password being known only to the researcher(s). As part of the ethical review of research, an important issue is safety of data within the organization. The Data Protection Officer or Caldicott Guardian must sign the research ethics approval form to indicate that he or she is satisfied that the requirements and arrangements comply with the Data Protection Act 1998. Indeed, the whole process of ethical review is concerned with protecting patients from potential harm resulting from their involvement in a research study.

The sponsoring company should never receive data with patients' names or codes that will help to identify individual patients; all data must be anonymized before it is submitted to the company for analysis.

Cooperate with others in the team

Teamwork is vital to the success of any care programme with each member having a discrete and important role to play. Each person, from porters, nurses, therapists, housekeeping services to consultants, has a valuable individual and collective contribution to make towards improving the patient experience of health care.

The importance of good documentation must not be underestimated to ensure continuity and high standards of care. Sharing reliable information about patients and clients underpins good health-care practice, and hence the need for timely, accurate and comprehensive recording.

Maintain your professional knowledge and competence

Health-care practitioners have a duty under clinical governance to maintain up-to-date knowledge and skills. Part of the duty of care of the practitioner is to deliver evidence-based patient care, based on sound research findings, where possible. This can be achieved only by life-long learning in whichever way suits the individual. Study days are useful provided that they are used as a reflective experience and the practitioner returns to practice motivated to experiment with new ways of working, with a deeper understanding of a subject or willing and able to enter into informed debate with colleagues about possible changes to practice. Drawbacks, often experienced by practitioners attending study days, include lack of funding and allocation of time. However, many of the wound care and equipment companies organize study days for practitioners, free of charge, around the country.

There is a plethora of excellent tissue viability books and journals readily available to buy and access in libraries (see under 'Local policies and resources'). The Internet provides an easier way to obtain information but requires access and searching skills (see under 'Local policies and resources'). The onus is on the practitioner to seek out information and use it appropriately in practice.

Be trustworthy

As with other fields of practice, that of wound care requires close collaboration and cooperation with industries such as the wound care product and bed and mattress industry. As a health-care practitioner, no preference for a single company, product or service must be demonstrated. Any financial or other interests must be declared and professional judgement must not be influenced by commercial considerations. Recommendations for treatments or products must be based on clinical appropriateness, evidence of efficacy and value for money, and in conjunction with the patient's preference.

Act to identify and minimize risk to patients and clients

All health-care practitioners must work together to provide a safe, therapeutic and ethical environment. If a patient is found to be adversely reacting to a dressing or therapy, a decision to discontinue must be quickly considered with other members of the team.

Managers should monitor training and ensure that practitioners are competent before carrying out tasks (competence is the possession of the skills and abilities required for lawful, safe and effective professional practice without direct supervision). It is the responsibility of the individual to access training in the use of new therapies and products before they are used, e.g. the application of vacuum-assisted closure (VAC) therapy to a difficult wound can be complex. No health-care practitioner should attempt to undertake practices for which they have not received training and been proved to be competent. The interests and safety of patients must prevail over everything else.

The number of complaints about the quality of basic nursing care is rising, particularly in relation to assessment, poor communication and inadequate documentation (Health Service Ombudsman or HSO 2002). The Essence of Care Benchmarking (Department of Health or DoH 2001b) exercise was introduced to try to rectify this deteriorating situation and re-focus practitioners back to considering and meeting the basic needs of patients.

Clinical governance and wound care

Clinical governance is a controls assurance function for the systems of clinical quality management. It makes acute trusts and primary care trusts accountable for the quality of clinical care provided and demands a fundamental change in attitude and culture within the NHS (DoH 1997). The primary aim of clinical governance is to re-establish the confidence and trust upon which the NHS is founded. There have been concerns about the quality of care that have attracted national publicity, public enquiries and a focus on failure. It is intended that clinical governance will support a process of continuous quality improvement throughout the NHS. Clinical governance sets out to ensure:

- that systems to monitor the quality of clinical practice are in place and functioning properly
- that clinical practice is reviewed and improved as a result
- that clinical practitioners meet standards such as those set out in 'good medical practice' issued by the General Medical Council (GMC).

Clinical governance aims to:

- restore public confidence
- restore professional image
- improve services – particularly the process of care
- respond to change.

Clinical governance provides a common purpose for clinical audit, research and development, risk management, quality, complaints, resources and education. It must be built on the good and effective systems already in place and integrated into the way things are done in the organization.

The implications for tissue viability are far-reaching in terms of guaranteeing high-quality care to the public and ensuring that the care is based on the best practice and scientific evidence available (Wilson 1999). Care provision must be satisfactory, consistent and responsive, with each practitioner responsible for the quality of his or her clinical and professional practice.

Questions for the organization

- Are we doing the right things?
- Are we doing things right?
- How will we know if we are doing things right?
- Do we have the capacity and capability?

A coordinated tissue viability service that encompasses all members of the multidisciplinary team is needed in every organization. The foundation for the service should comprise guidelines that steer towards best practice. Examples of useful evidence-based guidelines include the *Pressure Ulcer Risk Assessment and Prevention Clinical Guidelines* (National Institute for Clinical Excellence or NICE 2001) and *Pressure Ulcer Prevention Guidelines* (NICE 2003), with several more planned to address the problem of erratic wound care practice. They contain useful guidance about what activities should be pursued to prevent pressure ulcers occurring. Nationally developed guidelines provide evidence-based standards that can be incorporated into local policies, guidelines and protocols against which local practice may then be audited. Clinical audit is the means by which judgement of effectiveness is carried out. Audit of the quality of documentation, pressure ulcer incidence, use of equipment and dressings will provide information about the status of practice and indicate where improvements are needed. Clinical audit will be effective in improving the quality of care only if the audit loop is closed and re-evaluated, i.e. if changes are made and their impact measured repeatedly.

Litigation and best practice

Clinical practice is the most visible aspect in tissue viability and, therefore, subject to the most scrutiny when claims of medical negligence are made (Culley 2001). All patient records must be kept for a minimum of 8 years (even after death) to allow time for complaints/claims to be made. The most commonly cited cases in tissue viability are those concerning pressure injuries that are reported to have been awarded between £4000 and £12 500 (Tingle 1997). Recent personal involvement in a medico-legal case where a male patient suffered lower limb amputation as a result of pressure damage raised £100 000 in damages.

Before a complaint about health-care provision reaches court, it will have gone through several stages, during which time attempts will have been made to resolve the situation:

* local resolution
* independent review panel
* health service commissioner (Ombudsman).

If a case reaches court, the medical record is enlarged to poster size or put on a slide for all to view. Tiny errors become larger and inconsistencies are magnified. Medical record neatness, organization and completeness are critical. The basic principles of medical documentation fall into three main categories.

Professional risk of liability

Dual standards of care between wards in the same trust, which lead to different outcomes, can threaten the credibility and increase the liability of the whole organization. They can work to provide an argument for the plaintiff verdict. Variances must be avoided as far as possible. Standardization of practice demonstrates that the provider has thought about the issues and standards of care and can provide powerful evidence of optimum practice. It also shows that clinical professionals have addressed quality and safety issues in a proactive and reflective manner.

Clinical guidelines

Clinical guidelines are systematically developed statements designed to help practitioners and patients make decisions about appropriate health care for specific circumstances (Field and Lohr 1992). This means a recommendation for patient management that identifies one or more strategies for treatment – lawyers would concern themselves with the substance of the ideas and strategies that lie behind the label. The Department of Health actively promotes the development and use of guidelines: they provide a key vehicle for promoting evidence-based practice and a basis for systematic audit. Guidelines are fast becoming an increasing and established feature of the care environment. However, guidelines are not a substitute for clinical judgement.

Guidelines for pressure ulcer risk assessment and prevention were commissioned by the Department of Health and published by the NICE (2001). The guidelines were based on a systematic review carried out by the Royal College of Nursing, which revealed very little in the way of underpinning evidence for most practices undertaken to prevent pressure ulcers. However, the method used to develop the 2001 guidelines was an expert consensus group method. This means that a multidisciplinary group of experts in the field was convened to consider the evidence of clinical and cost-effectiveness found in the systematic review, and draw from their own and others' experience, to develop the guidelines.

National guidance is necessarily vague but sets the scene for health-care organizations to review their own arrangements in light of the guideline recommendations. Most organizations have locally developed policies, protocols or clinical guidelines to guide practice which take into consideration local resources, facilities, patient groups and staffing, but based on national recommendations. Guidelines, therefore, provide the standards against which practice should be measured.

Testing the theory

In law, a case will be judged against the prevailing clinical guidelines at the time of the incident, e.g. if a patient developed a pressure ulcer in 1991 the standard of nursing care would be judged against the clinical standard of 1991. An overview of what could have been expected at that time would be gained from expert witnesses. However, in wider-ranging general cases in law there will always be the basic standard to be achieved.

The Bolam principle is widely cited as the standard expected of the ordinary skilled person practising his or her skill, not the highest expert skill. This is the standard of care expected by the court as advised by the experts.

The Maynard test

Sometimes an opinion is rejected in court where there is a difference of medical opinion and, although one opinion will not be accepted as wrong, it will not constitute negligence. However, medicine is not an exact science and there are different ways of approaching problems. A guideline can protect a user but failure to follow a guideline would not mean an automatic finding of negligence. It would be good risk management practice to record the reason for not following the guideline.

Practice guidelines are simply one of many sources of evidence about what the standard of care should be in any given malpractice case. Failure to exercise clinical discretion could amount to negligent conduct. The court would be looking for the following:

- the development process of the guideline
- reasonableness of the guideline
- the information underpinning the guideline
- the quality of the research and clinical practice
- realism
- responsible minority medical opinion (the Bolam test); a tension exists between evidence-based and majority evidence-based practices and minority clinical practice founded on practice, precedent and experience, but not necessarily scientific evidence
- controlled environment of care – proactive and reflective approaches to problems.

Properly constructed and used guidelines have the potential to reduce complaints and litigation levels by improving channels of communication between health care and patients. The Medical Defence Union noted that 'a correlation has been demonstrated between poor communication and litigation'.

Implications for guideline developers

- Guidelines must be kept up to date because current cases will be judged against current accepted practice; long-standing cases will be judged against the 'gold standard' of the relevant time.
- Weeding out weak cases with guidelines is a reality.
- Improving the quality of care with guidelines as part of a risk management strategy.
- Guidelines could encourage lawyers to bring cases – plaintiff and defendant lawyers may use them.
- The danger of too many guidelines may provide scope for conflict.
- Guideline use will not result in increased legal exposure.

At the practical level, guidelines may be viewed as a framework within which practitioners can follow their own code of professional conduct (Bale and Jones 1997). The advantages associated with guidelines and protocols are summarized below.

Advantages (Bale and Jones 1997)

- should provide evidence-based (as far as possible) guidance
- provide a systematic framework in which practitioners can practise safely and confidently
- should ensure continuity of care for the patient
- should eliminate ritualistic practice and individual practitioner preferences
- encourage participation and contribution by all the team members during compilation
- provide a basis for evaluation of care through audit
- should be linked to the hospital/community formulary to maximize cost-effectiveness.

The disadvantages relate to the difficulties associated with convening a team and gaining their agreement, the time required for production and updating, and gaining widespread acceptance. Working to guidelines does, however, have the potential to reduce complaints and litigation, and can improve record-keeping and communication generally in health care.

Record-keeping that complies with established standards of care is a legitimate form of self-protection against litigation and can help when determining liability.

Appraising the wound management literature

Evidence-based practice is 'the process of systematically finding, appraising and using contemporaneous research findings as the basis for clinical decision-making' (Long and Harrison 1996). A more practical definition describes how it occurs: through the integration of clinical expertise with the best available external evidence from systematic research (Sackett 1997). The 'evidence' has been gathered to produce guidance for clinical practice, e.g. National Service Frameworks for diabetes, cancer, etc. with a focus on quality improvement rather than costs and throughput. Healthcare organizations are regularly monitored and regulated by the Commission for Healthcare Audit and Inspection (CHAI), using evidence-based standards to measure performance against clinical governance reviews.

As practitioners, we still have an individual responsibility to search for evidence and integrate what we find with our personal experience, and also to share and debate our conclusions with others. The following section offers guidance on how to read and appraise the research literature.

Reading research reports

There are many ways to read a research report; this is one suggestion in which the content has been drawn from several others.

First, the whole report should be read in order to establish an understanding of the content, context, aims, methods used and results. You may need to read it through a few times. Next, divide it into sections, and read and précis each separately to achieve full understanding and familiarity with the material, but do not forget the context of the whole text. Analyse each section, especially the conclusion. Form an overall impression of the clarity and style of the report and the relevance of the subject matter.

You are not setting out to be critical about the report; the intention is to evaluate the content and reflect on what use it can be to you. The good points as well as any bad points of the report should be described and, in particular, concentrate on the validity of the findings.

There are basically six parts to a research report; how they are arranged may vary and will depend on the style of the writer, nature of the study and purpose of the report:

1. introduction and background
2. a statement about the problem under investigation
3. review of the related literature
4. an explanation of the methodology, i.e. the research design and procedures used to conduct the research
5. an analysis of the data – results
6. discussion – interpretation of the findings on which the conclusions and recommendations are based.

The following checklist should guide your reading of a research report.

- **Introduction and background**
  - What is the study about?
  - Is there a summary or abstract?
  - Does the title indicate what the study is about?
  - Is the study experimental or descriptive in nature?
  - Is the work of interest to you or relevant to your work?
  - Why was the study carried out?
  - Was the purpose worthwhile?
  - Who asked for it?
  - Who paid for it?
  - How are the results to be used?
  - Is the report clearly presented, logical and well organized?

- **Problem statement**
  - Is the problem clearly defined?
  - Is the hypothesis or objective stated?
  - Are they derived from previous research?
  - Is the problem placed within the framework of existing theory or knowledge; is it clearly related to existing research?
  - Are definitions of the main concepts given and are they clear and concise?
  - Are any assumptions stated and are they justified?
  - Is it worth investigating?
  - Will it advance knowledge?

- **Review of the related literature**
  - Has any related research been carried out and is this clearly outlined?
  - Is the literature search comprehensive, up to date, well organized?
  - Does the literature suggest any tools or ideas relevant to the research?
  - Does it critically evaluate the literature?

- **Research design and methodology**
  - Where was the study undertaken?
  - What population is selected for the study?
  - How were the patients selected?
  - Does the method of sampling seem appropriate?
  - Is the sample large enough?
  - Is the sample representative of the population and unbiased?
  - Are any variables or factors pertinent to the study not included?
  - How is the information collected?
  - What instruments or tools are used?
  - Are examples included?

- How were the examples tested?
- Was there a pilot study?
- Are problems mentioned?
- Were the instruments used valid (i.e. did they measure what they were supposed to measure)?
- Were the instruments used reliable (i.e. could they be used again with the same kind of results)?
- Does the researcher take note of any ethical considerations?

• **Data analysis and interpretation**

- Are the data analysed by computer or by hand?
- Are appropriate statistical tests used?
- Has the author discussed each hypothesis/objective in the light of research findings/discussion?
- What are the main results of the study?
- Does the research meet the identified objectives?
- Was the hypothesis accepted or rejected?
- Are there any discrepancies between information presented in tables and graphs and that in the text of the article?
- Are the data clearly presented?
- What are the implications of the study?
- Is the discussion clearly related to the actual findings and the literature?
- Are the investigators' interpretations based on the data?
- Does the researcher discuss how much his or her findings can be generalized?
- Are suggestions made for further research?

• **Other questions to be answered may include**

- Is there an accurate reference and bibliography list?
- Are there details about the researcher?
- Is he or she qualified to do the research?
- Is it well written?

Critical appraisal of research is a learned skill.

Local policies and resources

Most health-care organizations will have pressure ulcer prevention policies, guidelines or protocols in operation to guide wound care practice; others will have wound care formularies. Each will set out what is expected in terms of best practice for each area of practice or wound type, cost-effective and effective options, and the availability of dressings and/or equipment. These documents are valuable learning resources for students to access up-to-date information.

The local tissue viability nurse, infection control nurse or equipment nurse is also an excellent source of information about tissue viability issues, including special arrangements for overweight patients. The internet has revolutionized access to information over the last few years, not least in the field of tissue viability. A recent Google search identified 647 000 sites relating to 'wound care', 130 000 for 'pressure sore' and 82 000 for 'pressure ulcer'. Much of this information has to be discounted as commercial, of unreliable source, out of date or questionable, because there is unfortunately no quality control. Unless the web address is known, much time and effort can be wasted searching blindly through thousands of irrelevant sites.

The following are recommended wound care sites:

- www.worldwidewounds.com: wound care articles and information
- www.tvna.org: Tissue Viability Nurses Association
- www.tvs.org.uk: Tissue Viability Society
- www.woundcaresociety.org: Wound Care Society
- www.ewma.org: European Wound Management Association
- www.epuap.org: European Pressure Ulcer Advisory Panel.

However, some of the commercial wound care and equipment sites do provide valuable information and educational material for practitioners that they might not otherwise be able to access. Examples include:

- Smith & Nephew Global Wound Academy: www.globalwoundacademy.com/us/index.asp
- 3M Healthcare: http://cms.3m.com/cms/GB/en/2-163/ilkluFY/view.jhtml
- Johnson & Johnson: www.jnjgateway.com/public/GBENG/6024ETHICON_Wound_Closure_Manual.pdf
- Huntleigh Healthcare: www.huntleigh-healthcare.co.uk/
- KCI Vacuum assisted therapy: www.kci1.com/woundmgmtrefguide.asp

Books on tissue viability

There have been several excellent tissue viability books written over the last few years. Some are listed below:

Bale S, Harding KG, Leaper D (2000) *An Introduction to Wounds*. London: EMAP Healthcare.

Bale S, Jones V (2000) *Wound Care Nursing. A patient-centred approach*, 2nd edn. London: Baillière Tindall.

Baranowski S, Ayello E (2003) *Wound Care Essentials: Practice principles*. London: Springhouse Publishing.

Bryant R (2000) *Acute and Chronic Wounds. Nursing management*, 2nd edn. London: Mosby.

Dealey C (2000) *The Care of Wounds*, 2nd edn. London: Blackwell Science.

Morison M, Moffatt C, Bridel-Nixon J, Bale S (1997) *The Management of Chronic Wounds*, 2nd edn. London: Mosby.

Sciarra J (2003) *Wound Care Made Incredibly Easy*. London: Lippincott, Williams & Wilkins.

Journals and supplements

The Journal of Tissue Viability – subscription with membership
Nursing Standard – quarterly tissue viability supplement
Nursing Times – quarterly tissue viability supplement
British Journal of Nursing – quarterly tissue viability supplement

Regular tissue viability articles can be found in:

Professional Nurse
Nurse2Nurse Magazine

This list is not exhaustive.

Study days

- The Tissue Viability Society hosts one conference a year.
- European Wound Management Association (EWMA) and European Pressure Ulcer Advisory Panel (EPUAP) hold annual conferences.
- Many companies hold study days around the UK or can be approached to organize a local study day or in-house training.
- Look in the nursing press for information about study days and conferences.

Are we getting it right for the future?

The discipline of tissue viability is becoming wider and deeper in terms of what is expected by managers and the general public. Health-care practitioners must be able to demonstrate that they are providing care that is underpinned by sound evidence in collaboration with colleagues, patients and their carers. Evidence of clinical effectiveness relating to providing the best possible care, in the right place, at the optimum time, and acknowledging the individuality of patients and their needs is essential.

Clinical benchmarking is becoming established as a useful tool for examining current clinical practice for comparison with what is currently considered to be best practice. The situation, however, is dynamic, because nursing, politics and the configuration of health services change over time. Education and life-long learning as principles of clinical governance are key to the process of improving health-care services.

Glossary of terms

Aerobic bacteria: Bacteria that thrive in an oxygen-rich environment.

Alginate: Dressings derived from seaweed to produce a hydrophilic gel on contact with exudate.

Alternating pressure mattress: Dynamic air mattress in which the cells alternately inflate and deflate to reduce interface pressure.

Anaerobic bacteria: Bacteria that thrive in an oxygen-free environment.

Angiogenesis: The production of new blood vessels in a wound – resulting in granulation tissue.

Antibacterial: A substance that kills or inhibits bacteria.

Antibiotic: A chemical substance that kills or inhibits bacteria.

Antimicrobial: A substance that destroys or prevents the growth of bacteria.

Assessment: Information obtained via observation, questioning, physical examination and clinical investigations to establish a baseline for planning care.

Autolysis: The body's natural capacity for breaking down necrotic tissue.

Blanching: Skin becomes paler when compression is applied as a result of local occlusion of capillaries.

Cellulitis: Inflammation and infection of the cells, associated with heat, redness, swelling and pain.

Chronic wound: A wound that has remained unhealed for more than 6 weeks.

Collagen: The most abundant protein in the body; found in bone, teeth, skin, hair, etc.

Contamination: Organisms present in wound exudate but not multiplying or clinically affecting the host.

Débridement: The removal of devitalized or contaminated tissue through surgery, larval therapy, autolysis or occlusive dressings.

Dehiscence: Separation of the opposed edges of a surgical wound.

Diabetic foot ulcer: Ulceration of the foot or lower leg as a result of underlying diabetic pathophysiology.

Emollients: A mixture of water with a suspension of oil usually with emulsifiers and preservatives.

Epithelialization: When a wound bed is level with the surface, epithelial cells will migrate over the wound to complete healing.

Erythema: Redness of the skin caused by inflammation or prolonged pressure.

Eschar: Hard necrotic tissue.

Evaluation: A critical appraisal or assessment; a judgement of the value, worth, character or effectiveness of interventions.

Excoriation: Where the skin has been traumatized – worn away or eroded as a result of incontinence or inappropriate dressings.

Exudate: Serous fluid that has passed through the walls of a damaged or overextended vein.

Factitious wound: A self-inflicted wound.

Fibroblast: In wound healing, fibroblasts stimulate cell migration, angiogenesis, embryonic development and healing.

Fistula: A passage that has formed between two organs, i.e. the bowel and the skin.

Gangrene: Devitalized, dead tissue caused by failure of the blood supply.

Granulation tissue: A complex combination of newly formed vascular tissues which lay down a matrix of cellular tissues during wound healing.

Growth factors: Cytokines and peptides vital for proliferation in wound healing.

Haematoma: A bruise or collection of blood in the tissues.

Haemostasis: The control of bleeding.

Homoeostasis: The body's natural mechanism for maintaining health constancy and ensuring survival.

Hydrogel: Water-based products for re-hydrating necrotic tissue.

Hydrophilic: Water loving – absorbent dressings.

Hydrophobic: Water hating – non-absorbent dressings.

Hypergranulation tissue (overgranulation): Excessive production of granulation tissue.

Inflammation: Natural defence against bacterial invasion; stimulates wound healing.

Interactive dressing: A dressing that mediates changes within the wound bed or fluid.

Ischaemia: Localized deficiency of arterial blood.

Laceration: A tearing or splitting of the skin caused by blunt trauma.

Leg ulcer: Wound of the lower limb that is frequently chronic in nature.

Maceration: The softening of tissue that becomes white and soggy after being moist or wet for a long time.

Macrophage: A phagocytic cell derived from the blood monocyte which plays a vital role in inflammation and initiates angiogenesis.

Malodour: Unpleasant odour from a wound.

Necrosis: Death of tissue or an organ in response to injury, disease or occlusion of blood flow.

Oedema: An unnatural accumulation of fluid in the interstitial spaces.

Pressure ulcer: An area of localized damage to skin and underlying tissue caused by pressure, shear, friction and/or a combination of these.

Pus: A product of inflammation usually caused by infection, containing used cells, debris and tissue elements.

Reactive hyperaemia: Observed as red flushing of skin following a period of occlusion and ischaemia.

Scab: Dried serous exudate after injury to the skin that has caused bleeding.

Septicaemia: Presence of pathogenic organisms or toxins in the bloodstream.

Sharp débridement: A method of débridement using scalpel or scissors to remove necrotic tissue.

Sinus: An epithelial cell-lined tube from the outside of the body to inside.

Slough: A mixture of dead white cells, dead bacteria, re-hydrated necrotic tissue and fibrous tissue.

Strike-through: Evidence of wound exudate appearing on the outside of the wound dressing indicating a need for dressing change.

Tissue viability: The ability of tissue to perform its normal function optimally.

Ulcer: A lesion of the skin which can be accompanied by necrotic tissue and caused by a number of factors.

Vasoconstriction: The arteries and arterioles constrict under the influence of drugs, hormones or cold.

Vasodilatation: The lumen of blood vessels opens and widens, blood flow slows, and more oxygen can reach the tissues.

Wound: A break in the epidermis that can be related to trauma or pathological changes within the skin or body.

This list is not exhaustive. Definitions are taken from Collins et al. (2002), Davis et al (1992) and Weller (2000).

References

Adam K, Oswald I (1983) Protein synthesis, body renewal and the sleep-wake cycle. Clinical Science 65: 6; 561–567.

Alderson M (1983) An Introduction to Epidemiology, 2nd edn. London: Macmillan.

Alterescu V, Alterescu M (1992) Pressure ulcers: assessment and treatment. Orthopaedic Nurse 11(2): 37–49.

Alvarez OM, Mertz PM, Smerbeck RV, Eaglstein WH (1983) The healing of superficial skin wounds is stimulated by external electrical current. Journal of Investigative Dermatology 81: 144–148.

Alvarez OM, Rozint J, Wiseman D (1989) Moist environment for healing: matching the dressing to the wound. Wounds 1(1): 35–51.

Anderson M (1995) Perceived distress in leg ulcer patients: questionnaire and preliminary findings. Quality of Life Research 4: 38–89.

Anthony DM (1987) Are you in the dark? Nursing Times 83(34): 24–26.

Anthony DM (1993) Measuring pressure sores and venous leg ulcers. Community Outlook 3(8): 35–37.

Arnold F (1996) Growth factor treatment for wounds: magic bullets or high tech hype? In: Cherry GW, Gottrup F, Lawrence JC, Moffatt CJ, Turner TD (eds), Proceedings of the 5th European Conference on Advances in Wound Management. London: Macmillan Magazines Ltd.

Ashcroft G, Horan MA, Ferguson MW (1997a) The effect of aging on wound healing: immunolocalisation of growth factors and their receptors in a murine incisional model. Journal of Anatomy 190: 351–365.

Ashcroft G, Dodsworth J, Van Boxtel E (1997b) Estrogen accelerates wound healing associated with an increase in TGF B1 levels. Nature and Medicine 3: 1209–1215.

Audit Commission (2000) Testing Times. A Review of the Diabetes Services in England and Wales. Audit Commission of England & Wales.

Baker SR, Stacey MC, Sing G et al. (1992) Aetiology of chronic leg ulcers. European Journal of Vascular Surgery 6: 245–251.

Bale S (1992) Wound dressings. In: Morison M, Moffatt C, Bridel-Nixon J, Bale S (eds), Nursing Management of Chronic Wounds. London: Mosby, pp. 103–118.

Bale S, Harding K, Leaper D (2000) An Introduction to Wounds. London: EMAP Ltd.

Bale S, Jones V (1997) Wound Care Nursing. A Patient-centred Approach. London: Baillière Tindall.

Bale S, Morison M (1997) Patient assessment. In: Morison M, Moffatt C, Bridel-Nixon J, Bale S (eds), Nursing Management of Chronic Wounds. London: Mosby, pp. 69–86.

219

Ballard K, Baxter H (2001) Promoting healing in static wounds. Nursing Times 97(14): 52.

Banwell PE (1999) Topical negative pressure therapy in wound care. Journal of Wound Care 8(2): 79–84.

Barbenel JC, Jordan MM, Nichol SM, Clark MO (1977) Incidence of pressure sores in the Greater Glasgow Health Board Area. Lancet ii: 548–550.

Barnett A (1992) Prevention and treatment of diabetic foot ulcers in diabetic patients in a multidisciplinary setting. Foot Ankle International 16: 388–394.

Barton A, Barton M (1981) The Management and Prevention of Pressure Sores. London: Faber & Faber.

Becker RO (1961) The bioelectric factors in amphibian limb regeneration. American Journal of Orthopaedics 43A: 643–656.

Becker GD (1986) Identification and management of the patient at high risk of wound infection. Head and Neck Surgery 8: 205–210.

Beedle D (1993) Beating the bug. Nursing Times 89(45 suppl): 2–4.

Bellamy K (1995) Photography in wound care. Journal of Wound Care 4: 313–316.

Benbow M (2000) Mixing and matching dressing products. Nursing Standard 14(49): 56–62.

Benbow M (2001) Assessing wounds. Practice Nurse 21(6): 44–50.

Benbow M, Iosson G (2002) Fistula management following an appendicectomy: nursing challenges. Journal of Wound Care 11(2): 59–61.

Benbow M, Iosson G (2004) A clinical evaluation of Urgotul to treat acute and chronic wounds. British Journal of Nursing 13(2): 105–9.

Berg RW (1988) Etiology and pathophysiology of diaper dermatitis. Advanced Dermatology 3: 75–98.

Bergstrom N, Braden B, Laguzza A (1987) The Braden Scale for predicting pressure sore risk. Nursing Research 36: 205–210.

Betts JA, Molan PC (2001) A pilot trial of honey as a wound dressing has shown the importance of the way honey is applied to wounds. Poster presentation, 11th Conference of the European Wound Management Association 2001, Dublin, Ireland.

Bevan J (1978) A Pictorial Handbook of Anatomy and Physiology. London: Mitchell Beazley.

Bibby BA, Collins BJ, Ayliffe GA (1986) A mathematical model for assessing risk of post-operative wound infection. Journal of Hospital Infection 8(1): 31–38.

Black PK (1995) Caring for large wounds and fistulas. Journal of Wound Care 4(1): 23–26.

Bliss M (1990) Editorial – preventing pressure sores. The Lancet 335: 1311–1312.

Bolton L, Pirone L, Chen J, Lydon M (1990) Dressings' effects on wound healing. Wounds 2: 126–134.

Bond C (1998) Eating matters – improving dietary care in hospitals. Nursing Standard 12(17): 41–42.

Borwell B (1994) Nursing management of the patient with a gastro-intestinal fistula. Journal of Tissue Viability 4(1): 23–26.

Bosanquet N (1992) Costs of venous ulcers: from maintenance therapy to investment programmes. Phlebology 7(suppl 1): 44–46.

Boulton AJM (1994) Diabetic medicine. Diabetic Medicine 11(1): 5.

Boulton AJM (1996) The pathogenesis of diabetic foot problems: an overview. Diabetic Medicine 13: S12–S17.

Boykin JV (2002) How hyperbaric oxygen therapy helps heal chronic wounds. Nursing 32(6): 24.

Braden B, Bergstrom N (1987) A conceptual schema for the study of the etiology of pressure sores. Rehabilitation Nursing 12(1): 8–16.

Bradley JM (1985) Methicillin resistant *Staphylococcus aureus* in a London hospital. The Lancet i: 1493–1495.

Bridel J (1993) The aetiology of pressure sores. Journal of Wound Care 2: 2308.

Bridel-Nixon JE (1997a) Pressure sores. In: Morison M, Moffatt C, Bridel-Nixon J, Bale S (eds), Nursing Management of Chronic Wounds. London: Mosby, pp. 153–176.

Bridel-Nixon JE (1997b) Other chronic wounds. In: Morison M, Moffatt C, Bridel-Nixon J, Bale S (eds), Nursing Management of Chronic Wounds. London: Mosby, pp. 221–224.

British Association of Dermatologists (1992) Dermatology – A Service Under Threat. A Position Paper. London: Schering Plough.

British Association of Dermatologists (1993) British Association of Dermatologists and Canadian Dermatology Association joint annual meeting abstracts. British Journal of Dermatology 129 Supp. 42: 17–70.

British Heart Foundation (1999) Peripheral Arterial Disease. Patient information book. London: British Heart Foundation.

British Heart Foundation (2001) Factfiles 09-2001. Peripheral vascular disease (www.bhf.org.uk/professionals/index).

Broussard CL, Mendez-Eastman S, Frantz R (2000) Adjuvant wound therapies. In: Morison M, Moffatt C, Bridel-Nixon J, Bale S (eds), Nursing Management of Chronic Wounds. London: Mosby, pp. 431–453.

Brown JAC (ed.) (2001) Pears Pocket Medical Encyclopaedia. London: Little, Brown & Co.

Bryant R (1987) Wound repair: a review. Journal of Enterostomal Therapy 14: 262–266.

Bryant R (1992) Skin. In: Bryant R (ed.), Acute and Chronic Wounds. Nursing management. London: Mosby Year Book, pp. 1–30.

Bucknole W (1996) Treating venous ulcers in the community. Journal of Wound Care 5: 258–260.

Bullen JJ, Cushnie GH, Stoner HB (1966) Oxygen uptake by *Clostridium welchii* type A: its possible role in environmental infections in passively immunised animals. British Journal of Experimental Pathology 47: 488.

Burnand KG, Whimster I, Naidoo A, Browse NL (1982) Pericapillary fibrin in the ulcer-bearing skin of the leg: the cause of lipodermatosclerosis and venous ulceration. British Medical Journal 285: 1071–1072.

Callam MJ, Ruckley CV, Harper DR, Dale JJ (1985) Chronic ulceration of the leg: extent of the problem and provision of care. British Medical Journal 290: 1855–1856.

Carroll R, Johnson L (1991) Using a wound assessment chart. Nursing Standard 11(special suppl) 5(25): 8–9.

Casewell MW (1995) New threats to the control of methicillin resistant *Staphylococcus aureus*. Journal of Hospital Infection 30(suppl): 465–471.

Castledine G (1992) Wound care: how well do you dress? British Journal of Nursing 1: 347–348.

Chaffrey R (1997) Case study: larval therapy for an infected insect bite. World Wide Wounds (www.smtl.co.uk.World-Wide-Wounds/1997/october/larvaltherapy/larvalcasestudy.html).

Chant A (1990) Tissue pressure, posture, and venous ulceration. Lancet 336: 1050–1051.

Cherry GW, Ryan T J (1996) Enhanced wound angiogenesis with a new hydrocolloid dressing. Royal Society of Medicine International Congress and Symposium Series 88: 5–14.

Cherry G, Dealey C, Lawrence JC, Turner TD (1998) Proceedings of the 6th European Conference on Advances in Wound Management. London: Macmillan.

Clark M (1994) The financial costs of pressure sores to the UK National Health Service. In: Cherry GW, Leaper DJ, Lawrence JC, Milward P (eds), Proceedings of the 4th European Conference on Advances in Wound Management, Copenhagen. London: Macmillan Magazines, pp. 48–50.

Clark M, Watts S (1994) The incidence of pressure sores within a national health service trust hospital during 1991. Journal of Advanced Nursing 20: 33–36.

Clinical Standards Advisory Group (1993) Prevention and Treatment of Pressure Sores – Guidelines for good practice. London: Middlesex University Health Research Centre.

Cobb A, Knaggs E (2003) The nursing management of enterocutaneous fistulae: a challenge for all. British Journal of Nursing 12(17): S32–S38.

Coleridge-Smith PD, Thomas P, Scurr JH, Dormandy JA (1988) Causes of venous ulceration: a new hypothesis. British Medical Journal 296: 1726–1727.

Collier M (1996) Leg ulceration: a review of causes and treatment. Nursing Standard 10(31): 49–51.

Collier M (1997) Know-how: a guide to vacuum assisted closure (VAC). Nursing Times 93(5): 32–33.

Collier M (1999) Pressure ulcer development and principles for prevention. Nursing and Residential Care 2(9): 67–68.

Collier M (2000) Preventing and managing pressure ulcers on heels. Nursing Times 96, (Supp. 29): 7–8.

Collier M (2002) Wound bed preparation. Nursing Times 98(2), NT Plus-Wound Care (suppl).

Collier M (2003) Understanding wound inflammation. Nursing Times 30(25): 63–64.

Collins F, Hampton S, White R (2002) A–Z Dictionary of Wound Care. Surrey: Quay Books.

Connor H (1994) Prevention of diabetic foot problems. In: Boulton AJM, Connor H, Cavanagh PR (eds), The Foot in Diabetes, 2nd edn. Chichester: John Wiley, pp. 126–134.

Cookson B (1998) The emergence of mupirocin resistance: a challenge to the infection control and antibiotic prescribing practice. Journal of Antimicrobial Chemotherapy 41(1): 11–18.

Cooper P, Gray D (1998) Skin integrity following incontinence: a randomised trial (oral presentation). Proceedings of the 9th European Wound Conference, Harrogate.

Cooper RA, Molan PC (1999) Honey in wound care. Journal of Wound Care 8(7): 340.

Cork MJ (1997) Simple, effective but underused. Community Pharmacy April: 269.

Cornwall JV, Dore CJ, Lewis J D (1986) Leg ulcers: epidemiology and aetiology. British Medical Journal 73: 693–696.

Coull F (2003) Surgical Wound Healing. Essential wound management for day-to-day practice. London: Medical Education Partnership.

Crawford M (1999) Emollients: treatment for dry skin disorders in older people. British Journal of Community Nursing 4: 269–274.

Crowcroft N, Maguire H, Fleming M, Peacock J, Thomas J (1996) Methicillin resistant *Staphylococcus aureus*. Journal of Hospital Infection 34: 301–309.

Cruse PJE, Foord R (1980) The epidemiology of wound infection. Surgical Clinics of North America 60: 27–40.

Cullen B (2001) Promogran – mode of action. Diabetic Foot 4(suppl 3): S4–S5.

Culley F (2001) The tissue viability nurse and effective documentation. British Journal of Nursing 10(suppl 15): S30–S39.

Cullum N, Deeks JJ, Fletcher AW, Sheldon TA, Song F (1995) Preventing and treating pressure sores. Quality Health Care 4: 289–97.

Cullum N, Nelson EA, Flemming K, Sheldon T (2001) Systematic reviews of wound care management (5) beds; (6) compression; (7) laser therapy, therapeutic ultrasound, electrotherapy and electromagnetic therapy. Health Technology Assessment 5(9): 1–221.

Cutting K (1994) Factors influencing healing. Nursing Standard 8(50): 33–36.

Cutting K (1996) Definition of terms. Journal of Wound Care Resource File. London: Macmillan Magazines Ltd.

Cutting K (1997) Wounds and evidence of infection. Nursing Standard 11(25): 49–52.

Cutting K (1998) Wounds and infection. Wound Care Society Educational Leaflet 5(2).

Cutting K, Harding K (1994) Criteria for identifying wound infection. Journal of Wound Care 3: 198–201.

Cuzzell RZ (1988) The new RYB color code. American Journal of Nursing 88: 1342–1346.

Dale J, Callam M, Ruckley CV, Harper DR, Berrey PN (1983) Chronic ulcers of the leg: a study of prevalence in a Scottish community. Health Bulletin (Edinburgh) 41: 310–314.

Danielson L, Cherry G, Harding K, Rollman O (1997) Use of Iodosorb/Iodoflex on venous leg ulcer colonised with *Pseudomonas aeruginosa*. In: Leaper DJ, Cherry G, Dealey C, Lawrence JC, Turner TD (eds), Proceedings of the 6th European Conference on Advances in Wound Management. London: Macmillan.

David JA, Chapman RG, Chapman RG, Lockett B (1983) An Investigation of the Current Methods used in Nursing for the Care of Patients with Established Pressure Sores. Northwick Park, Middlesex: Nursing Practice Research Unit.

Davis M, Dunkley P, Harden RM et al. (1992) The Wound Programme. Dundee: Centre for Medical Education.

Dealey C (1994) The Care of Wounds. Oxford: Blackwell Scientific Publications.

Dealey C (1999) Measuring the size of the leg ulcer problem in an acute trust. British Journal of Nursing 8: 850–852, 854, 856.

Dealey C (2000) The Care of Wounds. A Guide for Nurses. London: Blackwell Science.

Denham J (2000) All hospitals to monitor hospital acquired infection. Press release ref: 2000/0584. London: Department of Health.

Department of Health (1991) Health of the Nation. London: HMSO.

Department of Health (1993) Pressure Sores: A key quality indicator. London: Department of Health.

Department of Health (1996) MRSA – What nursing and residential homes need to know. London: Department of Health.

Department of Health (1997) The New NHS: Modern, dependable. London: The Stationery Office.

Department of Health (2000) UK Antimicrobial Resistance Strategy and Action Plan. London Department of Health.

Department of Health (2001a) National Service Framework for Diabetes (www.doh.gov.uk/nsf/diabetes/ch2/complications.htm).

Department of Health (2001b) The Essence of Care: Patient-focused benchmarking for health care practitioners. The Stationery Office. London.

Department of Health (2003) Specialised Services National Definitions Set, 2nd edn. Hyperbaric Oxygen Treatment Services (Adult) – Definition No 28 (www.doh.gov.uk/specialisedservicesdefinitions/28hyperbaric2nd.PDF).

Department of Trade and Industry (1999) Burns and Scalds. Accidents in the home. London: DTI (www.dti.gov.uk/homesafetynetworks/bs_intro.htm) last accessed 15/11/2003.

DeSaxe M, Cooke M, Mayon-White R, Galbraith NS (1983) Methicillin resistant *Staphylococcus aureus* in the UK. Communicable Disease Report CDR 83/86 9 September.

Deva AK, Siu C, Nettle WJ (1997) Vacuum assisted closure of a sacral pressure sore. Journal of Wound Care 6: 311–312.

Dickerson J (1995) The problem of hospital-induced malnutrition. Nursing Times 92(4): 44–45.

Dire DJ (1992) Emergency management of dog and cat bite wounds. Emergency Medicine Clinics of North America 10: 719–736.

Dormandy JA, Ray S (1996) The natural history of peripheral artery disease. In: Tooke JE, Lowe GDO (eds) Textbook of Vascular Medicine. London: Arnold, pp. 162–175.

Doughty B (1992) Principles of wound healing and wound management. In: Bryant R (ed.), Acute and Chronic Wounds. Nursing management. London: Mosby Year Book, pp. 31–68.

Doughty DB, Waldrop J, Ramundo J (2000) Lower extremity ulcers of vascular etiology. In: Bryant R (ed.), Acute and Chronic Wounds. Nursing management, 2nd edn. London: Mosby, pp. 265–300.

Draper J (1985) Making the dressing fit the wound. Nursing Times 81(4): 32–35.

Drugs and Therapeutics Bulletin (1991) Local applications to wounds 1. Cleansers, antibacterials, debriders. Drugs and Therapeutics Bulletin 29(24): 93–94.

Duckworth G, Heathcock R (1995) Guidelines on the control of methicillin resistant *Staphylococcus aureus* in the community. Journal of Hospital Infection 31: 1–42.

Dunk-Richards G (1985) Mortality of multi-resistant *Staphylococcus aureus*. Lamp 42(5): 52–64.

Dyson M (1995) Role of ultrasound in wound healing. In: McCulloch JM, Kloth LC, Feedar JA (eds), Wound Healing: Alternatives in management, 2nd edn. London: Davis. pp. 318–346.

Dyson M, Lyder C (2001) Wound management: physical modalities. In: Morison M (ed.), The Prevention and Treatment of Pressure Ulcers. London: Mosby, pp. 177–194.

Eaglstein WH (1985) Experiences with biosynthetic dressings. Journal of the American Academy of Dermatology 12: 434–440.

Editorial (1990) Management of smelly tumours. Lancet 335: 141–142.

Edmonds ME, Blundell M, Morris HE (1986) Improved survival of the diabetic foot: the role of the specialist foot clinic. Quarterly Journal of Medicine 232: 165–171.

Edmonds ME, Boulton A, Buckenham T et al. (1996) Report of the Diabetic Foot and Amputation Group. Diabetic Medicine 13(9 suppl 4): S27–S429.

Edwards J (2001) Managing burns effectively. Practice Nurse 12(9): 361–5.

Efem SE (1988) Clinical observations on the wound healing properties of honey. British Journal of Surgery 75: 679–681.

Elcoat C (1986) Stoma Care Nursing. London: Baillière Tindall.

Ellis DA, Shaikh A (1990) The ideal tissue adhesive in facial plastic and reconstructive surgery. Journal of Otolaryngology 19: 68–72.

Emmerson AM, Enstone JE, Griffin M, Kelsey MC, Smyth ET (1996) The Second National Prevalence Survey of infection in hospitals – overview of the results. Journal of Hospital Infection 32: 175–90.

European Pressure Ulcer Advisory Panel (1999) Pressure Ulcer Treatment Guidelines. Oxford: EPUAP.

European Pressure Ulcer Advisory Panel (2002) Summary report of pressure ulcer prevalence data collected across 5 European countries. Oxford: EPUAP.

Evans AJ (1975) The modern treatment of burns. British Journal of Hospital Medicine 13: 287.

Everett W (1985) Wound sinus or fistula. In: Westaby S (ed.), Wound Care. London: William Heineman Medical Books Ltd, pp. 84–90.

Exton-Smith AN (1971) Nutrition of the elderly. British Journal of Hospital Medicine 5: 639–645.

Faber WR, Michels PPJ, Maats B (1993) The neuropathic foot. In: Westerhot W (ed.), Leg Ulcers: Diagnosis and treatment. Amsterdam: Elsevier.

Fabian TS, Kaufman HJ, Lett ED et al. (2000) The evaluation of sub-atmospheric pressure and hyperbaric oxygen in ischaemic full-thickness wound healing. American Surgery 66: 1136–1143.

Fakhri O, Amin M (1987) The effect of low voltage electric therapy on the healing of resistant skin burns. Journal of Burn Care Research 8: 15.

Fakhry SM, Alexander J, Smith D (1995) Regional and institutional variations in burn care. Journal of Burn Care Rehabilitation 16: 86–90.

Falanga V, Marolis D, Alvarez O et al. (1998) Rapid healing of venous ulcers and lack of clinical rejection with an allogeneic cultured human skin equivalent. Archives of Dermatology 134: 293–300.

Faris I (1982) The Management of the Diabetic Foot. Edinburgh: Churchill Livingstone.

Ferguson A (1988) Best performer. Nursing Times 84(14): 525.

Field FK, Kerstein MD (1994) Overview of wound healing in a moist environment. American Journal of Surgery 167(1A): S2–S6.

Field MJ, Lohr KN (1992) Guidelines for Clinical Practice. From development to use. Washington DC: National Academy Press.

Finegold S (1982) Pathogenic anaerobes. Archives of Internal Medicine 142: 1988–1992.

Flanagan M (1989) Wound Care Society Educational Leaflet No 5.

Flanagan M (1993) Predicting pressure sore risk: a guide to the risk factors identified in the most common risk assessment scales. Journal of Wound Care 2: 215–2118.

Flanagan M (1994) Assessment criteria. Nursing Times 90(35): 76–88.

Flanagan M (1997a) Wound cleansing. In: Morison M, Moffatt C, Bridel-Nixon J, Bale S (eds), Nursing Management of Chronic Wounds. London: Mosby, pp. 87–102.

Flanagan M (1997b) The physiology of wound healing. In: Glover D, Miller M (eds) Wound Management: Theory and Practice. Edinburgh: Churchill Livingstone.

Flanagan M (1999) Reviewing the case for debridement. Journal of Wound Care 8: 267.

Flanagan M (2001) A practical framework for wound assessment 1: physiology. In: Ashurst S, Cruikshank J, Bradbury M (eds), Aspects of Skin and Wound Care Nursing, pp. 30–40. British Journal of Nursing monograph (e-book, www.quaybooks.com).

Flanagan M (2003) Improving accuracy of wound measurement in clinical practice. Ostomy Wound Management 49(10): 28–40.

Flanagan M, Graham J (2001) Should burn blisters be left intact or debrided? Journal of Wound Care 10(2): 41–45

Fleishman W, Strecker W, Bombelli M, Kinzl L (1993) Vacuum sealing as treatment of soft tissue damage in open fractures. Unfallchirug 96: 488–492. Cited by Thomas (2001).

Fletcher J (2001) How can we improve prevalence and incidence monitoring? Journal of Wound Care 10: 311–314.

Forrest S (2000) Assessing the risk of MRSA. Nursing Times 96(42): 39–40.

Foster A (1999) Diabetic ulceration. In: Miller M, Glover D (eds), Wound Management. Theory and Practice. London: NT Books, pp. 72–83.

Foulds I, Barker A (1983) Human skin battery potentials and their possible role in wound healing. British Journal of Dermatology 109: 515.

Fowkes FGR (1992) Smoking, lipids glucose intolerance and blood pressure as risk factors for peripheral atherosclerosis compared with ischaemic heart disease in the Edinburgh Artery Study. American Journal of Epidemiology 135: 331–340.

Fowkes FG, Housely E, Cawood EH et al. (1991) Edinburgh Artery Study: prevalence of asymptomatic and symptomatic peripheral artery disease in the general population. International Journal of Epidemiology 20: 384–392.

Franks PJ (2001) Health economics: the cost to nations. In: Morison M (ed.), The Prevention and Treatment of Pressure Ulcers. London: Mosby, pp. 47–54.

Franks PJ, Moffatt CJ, Connolly M et al. (1994) Community leg ulcer clinics: effect on quality of life. Phlebology 9: 83–86.

Friedman GD (1994) Primer of Epidemiology, 4th edn. New York: McGraw-Hill.

Friedman S, Su DWP (1982) Hydrocolloid occlusive dressing management of leg ulcers. Archives of Dermatology 120: 1329–1331.

Fuhrer MJ, Garber SL, Rintala DH, Clearman R, Hart KA (1993) Pressure ulcers in community-resident persons with spinal cord injury: prevalence and risk factors. Archives of Physical and Medical Rehabilitation 74: 1172–1177.

Galvin J (2002) An audit of pressure ulcer incidence in a palliative care setting. International Journal of Palliative Nursing 8: 214–221

Gelbart M (1999) Ancient and modern: the best of both. Nursing Times 94(45): 69–70, 73.

Gilchrist B (1989) Treating leg ulcers. Nursing Times Community Outlook 85(6 suppl): 25–26.

Gilchrist B (1993) Wound care. Studying by proxy. Nursing Times 89(25): 60.

Gilchrist B (1999) Wound infection. In: Miller M, Glover D (eds), Wound Management. Theory and practice. London: NT Books.

Gilchrist B, Morison M (1992) Wound infection In: Morison M, Moffatt C, Bridel-Nixon J, Bale S (eds), Nursing Management of Chronic Wounds. London: Mosby, pp. 53–68.

Gilchrist B, Reed C (1989) The bacteriology of chronic venous ulcers treated with occlusive hydrocolloid dressings. British Journal of Dermatology 121: 337–344.

Goodall S (2001) Risk factor assessment for patients with peripheral arterial disease. Professional Nurse 17: 27–30.

Goodall B, Tomkins D S (1994) Nursing homes act as reservoir. British Medical Journal 308: 58.

Gordon M, Goodwin CW (1997) Initial assessment, management and stabilisation. Nursing Clinics of North America 32: 237–249.

Gould D (1987) Infection and Patient Care, A Guide for Nurses. London: Heinemann Nursing.

Gowar JP, Lawrence JC (1995) The incidence, causes and treatment of minor burns. Journal of Wound Care 4: 71–74.

Greenhalgh D (1996) The role of growth factors in wound healing. Journal of Trauma 41: 159–167.

Grey JE, Lowe G, Bale S, Harding KG (1998a) The use of Dermagraft in the treatment of long-standing and difficult to heal diabetic foot ulcers. In: Leaper DJ, Cherry G, Cockbill S et al. (eds), Proceedings of the EWMA/Journal of Wound Care, Spring Meeting: New Approaches to the Management of Chronic Wounds. London: Macmillan Magazines Ltd.

Grey JE, Lowe G, Bale S, Harding KG (1998b) The use of cultured dermis in the treatment of diabetic foot ulcers. Journal of Wound Care 7: 324–325.

Grocott P (1995a) The palliative management of fungating malignant wounds. Journal of Wound Care 4: 240–242.

Grocott P (1995b) Assessment of fungating malignant wounds. Journal of Wound Care 4: 333–336.

Haalboom JR (1991) The costs of decubitus. Nederlands Jijdschrift voor Geneeskunde 135: 606–610.

Haalboom JR (2000) The treatment or palliative care of pressure ulcers (www. internurse.com/tissueviab/march_2000/v6_art2.html, last accessed July 2003).

Haisfield-Wolfe ME, Rund C (1997) Malignant cutaneous wounds: a management protocol. Ostomy Wound Management 43(1): 56–66.

Haley RW (1991) Methicillin resistant *Staphylococcus aureus*. Annals of Internal Medicine 114: 162–164.

Ham R, Cotton L (1991) Limb Amputation. London: Chapman & Hall.

Hamer C, Roe B (1994) Patients' perceptions of chronic leg ulcers. Journal of Wound Care 3: 2: 99–101.

Hampton S (1997) Reliability in reporting pressure sore incidence. Professional Nurse 12: 627–630.

Hampton S (1999) Choosing the right dressing. In: Miller M, Glover D (eds), Wound Management. Theory and practice. London: NT Books, pp. 116–128

Hampton S, Collins F (2001) Keeping skin healthy: problems and solutions. Nursing and Residential Care 3: 210–213.

Harding KG (1996) Managing wound infection. Journal of Wound Care 5: 391–392.

Harris A, Rolstad BS (1992) Hypergranulation tissue: a non-traumatic method of management. In: 3rd European Conference on Advances in Wound Management Proceedings. London: Macmillan Magazines.

Hartnett JM (1998) Use of vacuum assisted wound closure in three chronic wounds. Journal of Wound Ostomy Continence Nursing 25: 281–90.

Hasdai D, Garratt KN, Grill DE, Lerman A, Holmes DR Jr (1997) The effect of smoking status on the long term outcome after successful percutaneous revascularisation. New England Journal of Medicine 336: 755–761.

Hauben D (1985) The evolution of wound healing by first intention: (a short history of wound treatment). Koroth 8(11–12): 77–88.

Haughton W, Young T (1995) Common problems in wound care: malodorous wounds. British Journal of Nursing 4: 959–960, 962–963.

Haury B, Rodeheaver G, Vensko J, Edgerton M, Edlich R (1980) Debridement: an essential component of traumatic wound care. In: Hunt T (ed.), Wound Healing and Wound Infection. New York: Appleton-Century Crofts, pp. 229–241.

Health Service Ombudsman (2002) HSC Investigations completed. December 2001. London: HSO.

Hecker B, Carron H, Schwartz D (1985) Pulsed galvanic stimulation: effects of current frequency and polarity on blood flow in healthy subjects. Archives of Physical Medicine and Rehabilitation 66: 369.

Herlihy B, Maebius (2000) The Human Body in Health and Illness. London: WB Saunders Co.

Hibbs (1988) Pressure Area Care. London: City and Hackney Health Authority.

Higley HR, Ksander GA, Gerhardt CO, Falanga V (1995) Extravasation of macromole-
cules and possible trapping of transforming growth factor-beta in venous ulceration.
British Journal of Dermatology 132: 79–85.

Hillstrom L (1988) Iodosorb compared to standard treatment in chronic venous leg
ulcers – a multi-centre trial. Acta Chirurgica Scandinavica Supplementum 554: 53–56.

Hofman D, Ryan TJ, Arnold F et al. (1997) Pain in venous leg ulcers. Journal of Wound
Care 6: 222–224.

Hohn D, Ponce B, Burton RW, Hunt TK (1977) Antimicrobial systems of the surgical
wound: A comparison of oxidative metabolism and microbiocidal capacity of phagocytes from wounds and from peripheral blood. American Journal of Surgery 133:
597–600.

Hollinworth H, Kingston JE (1998) Using a non-sterile technique in wound care.
Professional Nurse 13: 2269.

Hospital Infection Society (1998) Revised guidelines for the control of methicillin resistant Staphylococcus aureus infection in hospitals. Journal of Hospital Infection 39:
253–290.

Housley E (1988) Treating claudication in five words. British Medical Journal 296:
1483–1484.

Hughes A (1989) Nursing. In: Allbut C (ed.), A System of Medicine. London:
Macmillan, p. 433.

Hutchinson J (1992) Influence of occlusive dressings on wound microbiology: interim
results of a multi-centre trial of an occlusive hydrocolloid dressing. In: Harding K et
al. (eds), Proceedings of the First European Conference on Advances in Wound
Management. London: Macmillan.

Hutchinson JJ, Lawrence JC (1991) Wound infection under occlusive dressings. Journal
of Hospital Infection 17: 83–94.

Hyland ME, Ley A, Thomson B (1994) Quality of life of leg ulcer patients: questionnaire and preliminary findings. Journal of Wound Care 3(6): 29–48.

Irvin TT (1981a) Wound infection. In: Irvin TT (ed.), Wound Healing: Principles and
practice. London: Chapman & Hall, pp. 64.

Irvin TT (1981b) Wound Healing: Principles and practice. London: Chapman & Hall.

Irvin TT, Vassilikas JS, Chattopadhyay DK, Greaney MG (1978) Abdominal healing in
jaundiced patients. British Journal of Surgery 65: 521–522.

Jeter KF, Tintle TE, Chariker M (1990) Managing draining wounds and fistulas: new
and established methods. In: Krasner D (ed.), Wound Care: A clinical source book
for health professionals. King of Prussia, PA: Health Management Publications, pp.
240–246.

John C (2003) Focusing on Asian diabetes (http://news.bbc.co.uk/2/hi/health/
3261929.stm – last accessed 28 December 2003).

Jones V (1998) Debridement of diabetic foot lesions. Diabetic Foot 1(3): 88–94.

Jones V, Gill D (1998) Hydrocolloid dressings and diabetic foot lesions. Diabetic Foot
1(4): 127–134.

Junqueira I C, Carneiro J, Contopolus A (1977) Basic Histology, 2nd edn. Canada:
Lange Medical Publications.

Kakibuchi M, Hosokawa K, Fujikawa M, Yoshikawa K (1996) The use of cultured epidermal sheets in skin grafting. Journal of Wound Care 5: 487–490.

Kaltenthaler E, Whitefield M, Walters S, Akenhurst R, Paisley S (2001) UK, USA and
Canada: how do their pressure ulcer prevalence and incidence data compare?
Journal of Wound Care 10: 530–536.

Kiernan M (1997) Infected wounds: diagnosis and treatment. Practice Nursing August 8: 13.

Kindlen S, Morison M (1997) The physiology of wound healing. In: Morison M, Moffatt C, Bridel-Nixon J, Bale S (eds), Nursing Management of Chronic Wounds. London: Mosby, pp. 1–26.

Knowles A (1993) How to care for foot ulcers in people with diabetes. Diabetic Nurse 3(2): 68.

Krahn LE (2003) Factitious disorder: what to do when someone plays sick. Current Psychiatry On-line 2 (www.currentpsychiatry.com/2003_02/0203_factitious.asp).

Kumar P, Clark M (eds) (2001) Clinical Medicine, 4th edn. London: WB Saunders.

La Van F, Hunt TK (1990) Oxygen and wound healing. Clinics in Plastic Surgery 3: 463–472.

Lacey RW, Catto A (1993) Action of povidone-iodine against methicillin sensitive and resistant cultures of *Staphylococcus aureus*. Postgraduate Medical Journal 69(suppl 3): 78–83.

Laing W (1992) Chronic Venous Diseases of the Leg. London: Office of Health Economics.

Langemo DK, Melland H, Hanson D, Olson B, Hunter S (2000) The lived experience of having a pressure ulcer: a qualitative analysis. Advances in Skin and Wound Care 13: 225–235.

Lawrence J (1981) Burns: causes, management and consequences. Nursing 26: 1123–1125.

Lawrence JC (1994) Dressings and wound infection. American Journal of Surgery 167: S215–S245.

Lawrence JC (1997) Wound irrigation. Journal of Wound Care 6(1): 23–26.

Layton MC, Shareholder WJ Jr, Patterson JE (1995) The evolving epidemiology of methicillin resistant *Staphylococcus aureus*. Infection Control and Hospital Epidemiology 16(1): 12–17.

Leaper D (2000) History of wounds and the healing process. In: Bale S, Harding K, Leaper D (eds), An Introduction to Wounds. London: EMAP Healthcare, pp. 3–14.

Lees TA, Lambert D (1992) Prevalence of lower limb ulceration in an urban health district. British Journal of Surgery 79: 1032–4.

Leigh DA (1981) An eight year study of post-operative wound infection in two district general hospitals. Journal of Hospital Infection 2: 207–217.

Levett D, Smith S (2002) Survey of pressure ulcer prevalence in nursing homes. Elderly Care 12: 12–16.

Leyden JJ (1986) Diaper dermatitis. Dermatologic Clinics 4(1): 23–28 .

Lineaweaver W, Howard R, Soucy D et al. (1985) Topical antimicrobial toxicity. Archives of Surgery 120: 267–270.

Lippert H (1999) Compendium: Wounds and wound management. Heidenheim: Paul Hartmann.

Lipsett A (2003) www.guardian.co.uk/international/story/0,3604,1086566,00.html (last accessed 28th Dec 2003).

Lloyd N, Moody M (1999) Skin care for incontinent patients. Nursing and Residential Care 1(9): 15–17.

Locksley RM (1982) Multiple antibiotic resistance *Staphylococcus aureus*: introduction, transmission and evolution of nosocomial infection. Annals of Internal Medicine 97: 317–324.

Long A, Harrison S (1996) Evidence-based decision-making. Health Service Journal 106: 111.

Lookingbill DP, Marks JG (1993) Principles of Dermatology. London: WB Saunders Co.

McCallon SK, Knight CA, Valiulus JP, Cunningham MW, McCulloch JM, Farinas LP (2000) Vacuum-assisted closure versus saline-moistened gauze in the healing of postoperative diabetic foot wounds. Ostomy Wound Management 46:(8): 28–32, 34.

McGrath J, Schofield O (1990) Treatment of excessive granulation tissue with EMLA cream and 95% silver nitrate pencils. Clinical and Experimental Dermatology 15: 468.

McInerney RJ (1990) Honey – a remedy rediscovered. Journal of the Royal Society of Medicine 83: 127.

McSweeney P (1994) Assessing the cost of pressure sores. Nursing Standard 8(52): 25–26.

McWhirter JP, Pennington C (1994) Incidence and recognition of malnutrition in hospital. British Medical Journal 308: 945–948.

Maier SF, Laudenslager M (1985) Stress and health: exploring the links. Psychology Today 19(8): 44–49.

Mant AK (1985) Some medico-legal aspects of wounds. In: Westaby S (ed.), Wound Care. London: William Heinemann Medical Books Ltd, pp. 190–200.

Marhle G, Wemmer U, Matthies C (1989) Optimized intermittent topical treatment of eczema with fluprednidine. Zeitschrift für Hautkrankenheiren 64: 9. Cited by Crawford (1999).

Marks J, Harding KG, Hughes LE (1985) Pilonidal sinus excision: healing by open granulation. British Journal of Surgery 72: 637–640.

Martens MG, Kolrud BL, Faro S, Maccato M, Hammill H (1995) Development of wound infection or separation after Caesarian delivery: Prospective evaluation of 2431 cases. Journal of Reproductive Medicine 40: 171–175.

Martini FH, Bartholomew EF (2000) Essentials of Anatomy and Physiology, 2nd edn. Englewood Cliffs, NJ: Prentice Hall.

Mayfield JA, Reiber GE, Sanders LJ, Janisse D, Pogach LM (1998) Preventive foot care in people with diabetes. Diabetes Care 21: 2161–77.

Meers PD (1981) Report on the national survey of infection in hospitals. Journal of Hospital Infection 2: S29–S34.

Meers PD, Leong KY (1990) The impact of methicillin and aminoglycoside resistant *Staphylococcus aureus* on the pattern of hospital acquired infection in an acute hospital. Journal of Hospital Infection 16: 231–239.

Meers PD, Ayliffe GAJ, Emmerson AM et al. (1980) Report on the national survey of infection in hospitals. Journal of Hospital Infection 2(suppl): 29–34.

Mertz P, Eaglstein W (1984) The effect of a semi-occlusive dressing on the microbial population in superficial wounds. Archives of Surgery 119: 287–289.

Miller M, Dyson M (1996) The Principles of Wound Care. London: Macmillan Magazines Ltd.

Miller P, Powell D (1995) Developing wound evaluation tools. Nursing Standard 9(40): 25–27.

Mishriki SF, Law DJW, Jeffery PJ (1990) Factors affecting the incidence of post-operative wound infection. Journal of Hospital Infection 16: 223–230.

Moffatt C, Franks PJ, Oldroyd M et al. (1992) Community clinics for leg ulcers and impact on healing. British Medical Journal 305: 1389–1392.

Molan P (2001) Honey as a topical antibacterial agent for treatment of infected wounds (www.worldwidewounds.com/2001/november/Molan/honey-as-topical-agent.html).

Monteiro JA (1995) Human and animal bite wound infections. European Journal of Internal Medicine 6: 209–215.

Moody M, Grocott P (1993) Let us extend our knowledge base: assessment and management of fungating wounds. Professional Nurse 8(9): 58–79.

Morgan D (1993) Is there still a role for antiseptics? Journal of Tissue Viability 3(3): 80–84.

Morgan D (1997) Formulary of Wound Management Products, 7th edn. Surrey: Euromed Communications.

Morgan D (2000) Developing a formulary for wound dressings. Community Nurse 6(11): 37–8, 41.

Morison M (1988) Wound assessment. Professional Nurse 2: 315–317.

Morison M (1992a) A Colour Guide to the Nursing Management of Wounds. London: Wolfe Publishing.

Morison M (1992b) Wound care. Nursing Standard 6(37): 9–16.

Morison MJ, Moffatt CJ (1994) A Colour Guide to the Assessment and Management of Leg Ulcers, 2nd edn. London: Mosby.

Morison MJ, Moffatt CJ (1997) Leg ulcers. In: Morison M, Moffatt C, Bridel-Nixon J, Bale S (eds), Nursing Management of Chronic Wounds. London: Mosby, pp. 177–220.

Moro ML, Carrieri MP, Tozzi AE, Lana S, Greco D (1996) Risk factors for surgical wound infections in clean surgery: a multi-centre study. Italian PRINOS Study Group. Annals of Italian Chirugia 67: 13–19.

Mortimer P (1993) Skin problems in palliative care. In: Doyle D, Hanks G, Macdonald N (eds), Oxford Textbook of Palliative Medicine. Oxford: Oxford Medical Publications.

Moscati RM, Reardon RF, Lerner EB, Mayrose J (1998) Wound irrigation with tap water. Academic Emergency Medicine 5: 1076–1080.

Mullner T, Mrkonjic L, Kwasny O, Vecsei V (1997) The use of negative pressure to promote the healing of tissue defects: a clinical trial using the vacuum sealing technique. British Journal of Plastic Surgery 50: 194–199.

Murray J Boulton A (1995) The pathophysiology of diabetic foot ulceration. Clinical Podiatric Medical Surgery 12: 1–17.

Murray-Leisure KA, Geib S, Gracely D (1990) Control of methicillin resistant Staphylococcus aureus. Infection Control 11: 343–350.

National Burn Care Review (2001) Standards and Strategy for Burn Care in the British Isles. Manchester: British Association of Plastic Surgeons.

National Institute for Clinical Excellence (2001) Inherited Guideline B. Pressure ulcer risk assessment and prevention. London: NICE.

National Institute for Clinical Excellence (2003) Pressure Ulcer Prevention. Clinical guideline 7. London: NICE.

Naylor W (2001) Using a new foam dressing in the care of fungating wounds. British Journal of Nursing 10(6): 24–31.

Ndayisaba G, Bazira L, Habonimana E, Muteganya D (1993) Clinical and bacteriological outcome of wounds treated with honey. Journal of Orthopaedic Surgery 7: 202–204.

Nelson EA (1995) Management of leg ulcers. In: Kenrick M, Luker K (1995) Clinical Nursing Practice in the Community. London: Blackwell Science, pp 70–85.

Nelson A (2000) Accurate documentation in wound care. Nursing Times Supplement (Wound Care) 96(4): 10–11.

Nelzen O, Bergqvist D, Linghagen A (1991) Leg ulcer aetiology: a cross-sectional population study. Journal of Vascular Surgery 14: 5457–5464.

Newton H, Trudgian J, Gould D (2000) Expanding tissue viability practice through telemedicine. British Journal of Nursing 9(19): 42–48.

Nicholls R (1990) Leg ulcers: a study in the community. Nursing Standard 3(7 suppl): 4–6.

Nienhuijs SW, Manupassa R, Strobbe LJA, Rosman C (2003) Can topical negative pressure be used to control complex enterocutaneous fistulae? Journal of Wound Care 12: 343–345.

Niinikoski J, Grislis G, Hunt TK (1972) Respiratory gas tensions and collagen in infected wounds. Annals of Surgery 175: 588.

Nixon J, McGough A (2001) Principles of patient assessment: screening for pressure ulcers and potential risk. In: Morison M (ed.), The Prevention and Treatment of Pressure Ulcers. London: Mosby, pp. 55–74.

Nursing and Midwifery Council (2002a) An NMC Guide for Students of Nursing and Midwifery. London: NMC.

Nursing and Midwifery Council (2002b) Code of Professional Conduct. London: NMC.

Nyquist R, Hawthorn PJ (1987) The prevalence of pressure sores in an area health authority. Journal of Advanced Nursing 12: 183–187.

O'Dea K (1999) Prevalence of pressure damage in hospital patients in the United Kingdom. Journal of Wound Care 2: 221–225.

O'Toole EA, Goel MG, Lind FG (1997) hydrogen peroxide inhibits human keratinocyte migration. Dermatology Surgery 22: 315–322.

Oliver L (1997) Wound cleansing. Nursing Standard 11(20): 47–51.

Olsen DP (1992) Controversies in nursing ethics: a historical review. Journal of Advanced Nursing 17: 1020–1027.

Olsen B, Hanson D, Burd C, Savvage TR (1992) Pressure ulcer prevalence and incidence in a rehabilitation hospital. Rehabilitation Nurse 17: 341–345.

Papantonio CJ, Wallop JM, Kolodner KB (1994) Sacral ulcers following cardiac surgery: incidence and risk factors. Advances in Wound Care 7(2): 24–36.

Parker L (2000) Applying the principles of infection control to wound care. British Journal of Nursing 9: 394–398.

Patey DH, Fergusen JHL, Exley MD (1946) Gravity drainage in the prone position in the treatment of digestive fistulae of the abdominal wall. British Medical Journal 30: 814–815.

Pavillard ER, Wright EA (1957) An antibiotic from maggots. Nature 180: 916–917.

Pennels C (2001) The art of recording patient care information. Professional Nurse 16: 1359–1361.

Phillips L (2000) Cost-effective strategy for managing pressure ulcers in critical care: a prospective, non-randomised, cohort study. Journal of Tissue Viability 10: 2–6.

Pinchkofsky-Devin G (1994) Nutritional wound healing. Journal of Wound Care 3: 231–234.

Popp AJ (1995) Crossroads at Salerno: Eldridge Campbell and the writings of Teodorico Borgognoni on wound healing. Journal of Neurosurgery 83: 174–179.

Prete P (1997) Growth effects of *Phaenicia sericata* larval extracts on fibroblasts: mechanism for wound healing by maggot therapy. Life Sciences 60: 505–510.

Price P, Harding K (1996) Measuring health related quality of life in patients with chronic leg ulcers. Wounds 8(3): 914.

Pringle W (1995) The management of patients with enterocutaneous fistulae. Journal of Wound Care 4: 211–213.

Pudner R (1997) Wound cleansing. Journal of Community Nursing 11: 306.

Rainey J (2002) A Handbook for Community Nurses: Wound care. London: Whurr Publishers.

Ramundo J, Wells J (2000) Wound debridement. In: Bryant R (ed.), Acute and Chronic Wounds. Nursing management, 2nd edn. London: Mosby.

Ranaboldo CJ, Rowe-Jones DC (1992) Closure of laparotomy wounds: skin staples versus sutures. British Journal of Surgery 79: 1172–1173.

Rinseina W (1990) cited by Borwell B (1994) Collostomies and their management. Nursing Standard 8(45): 49–56.

Rinseina W (1992) Gastro-intestinal fistulas: management and results of treatment. Datawyse. Maastricht 149–152.

Rintala DH (1995) Quality of life considerations. Advances in Wound Care 8(4): 28–71, 28–83.

Robson MC, Stenberg BD, Heggers JP (1990) Wound healing alterations caused by infection. Clinical Plastic Surgery 17(3): 485–492.

Rodeheaver GT (1994) Conflicting points of view regarding the use of povidone-iodine. Ostomy Wound Management 40(8): 6.

Rolstad BS, Bryant RA (2000) Management of drain sites and fistulas. In: Bryant R (ed.), Acute and Chronic Wounds. Nursing management, 2nd edn. St Louis, MO: Mosby, pp. 317–341.

Rowell LB (1986) Human Circulation: Regulation during physical stress. Oxford: Oxford University Press.

Royal College of Nursing (1998) The Management of Patients with Venous Ulcers. Clinical Practice Guidelines. York: RCN Institute.

Ruckley CV, Dale JJ, Callam MJ et al. (1982) Causes of chronic leg ulcers. The Lancet ii: 615–616.

Russell AD, Hugo WB, Ayliffe GAJ (1982) Principles and Practice of Disinfection, Preservation and Sterilisation. London: Blackwell Scientific Publications.

Sackett DL (1997) Evidence-based medicine and treatment choices. The Lancet 349: 570.

Saltz R, Zamora S (1998) Tissue adhesives and applications in plastic and reconstructive surgery. Aesthetic Plastic Surgery 22: 439 –443.

Salzberg CA, Cooper-Vastola SA, Perez F, Viehbeck MG, Byrne DW (1995) The effects of non-thermal pulsed electromagnetic energy on wound healing of pressure ulcers in spinal cord-injured patients: a randomized, double-blind study. Ostomy Wound Management 41(3): 42–48.

Sciarra J (2003) Wound Care Made Incredibly Easy. London: Lippincott, Williams & Wilkins.

Selwyn S (1981) The topical treatment of skin infections. In: Maibach H, Aly R (eds), Skin Microbiology: Relevance to clinical infection. New York: Springer Verlag.

Sherman RA, Wyle F, Vulpe M (1995) Maggot debridement therapy for treating pressure ulcers in spinal cord injury patients. Journal of Spinal Cord Medicine 18: 71–74.

Sherman RA, Tran JM-T, Sullivan R (1996) Maggot therapy for venous stasis ulcers. Archives of Dermatology 132: 254–256.

Shubert V, Heraud J (1994) The effects of pressure and shear on skin microcirculation in elderly stroke patients lying in supine or semi-recumbent positions. Age and Aging 23: 405–410.

Siana JE, Frankild BS, Gottrup F (1992) The effect of smoking on tissue function. Journal of Wound Care 1(2): 37–41.

Simon HK, McLario DJ, Bruns TB, Zempsky WT, Wood RJ, Sullivan KM (1997) Long-term appearance of lacerations repaired using a tissue adhesive. Pediatrics 99: 193–195.

Sims R, Fitzgerald V (1985) Community Nursing Management of Patients with Ulcerating/fungating Breast Disease. London: Royal College of Nursing.

Sleigh JW, Linter SPK (1985) Hazards of hydrogen peroxide. British Medical Journal 291: 1706.

Smith PF, Meadowcroft AM, May DB (2000) Treating mammalian bite wounds. Journal of Clinical Pharmacy and Therapeutics 25: 85–99.

Spittle M, Collins RJ, Connor H (2001) The incidence of pressure sores following lower limb amputations. Practical Diabetes International 18: 57–61.

Starley IF, Mohammed P, Bickler SW (1999) The treatment of paediatric burns using topical papaya. Burns 25: 636–639.

Stemmer R (1969) Ambulatory elasto-compressive treatment of the lower extremities particularly with elastic stockings. Der Kassenatz 9: 1–8.

Stubbs (1989) Taste changes in cancer patients. Nursing Times 85(3): 49–50.

Subrahmanyam M (1993) Impregnated gauze versus polyurethane film (Opsite) in the treatment of burns – a prospective randomised study. British Journal of Plastic Surgery 46: 322–333.

Subrahmanyam M (1996) Honey dressing versus boiled potato peel in the treatment of burns: a prospective randomised trial. Burns 22: 491–493.

Sussman C, Dyson M (1998) Therapeutic and diagnostic ultrasound. In: Sussman C, Bates-Jensen BM (eds), Wound Care: A collaborative manual for physical therapists and nurses. New York: Aspen Publishers, pp. 427–445.

Tang AT, Ohri SK, Haw MP (2000a) Novel application of vacuum assisted closure technique to the treatment of sternotomy wound infection. European Journal of Cardiothoracic Surgery 17: 482–4.

Tang AT, Ohri SK, Haw MP (2000b) Vacuum assisted closure to treat deep sternal wound infection following cardiac surgery. Journal of Wound Care 9: 229–30.

Tanj LF, Phillips TJ (2001) Skin problems in the elderly. Wounds 13(3): 93–97.

Tatnall FM, Leigh IM, Gibson JR (1990) Comparative study of antiseptic toxicity on basal keratinocytes, transformed human keratinocytes and fibroblasts. Skin Pharmacology 3: 157–163.

Terrill PJ, Kedwards SM, Lawrence (1991) The use of Gore-tex bags for hand burns. Burns 17: 161–165.

Thomas S (1990) Wound Management and Dressings. London: The Pharmaceutical Press.

Thomas S (1992) Current Practices in the Management of Fungating Lesions and Radiation Damaged Skin. Bridgend, Glamorgan: The Surgical Materials Testing Laboratory.

Thomas S (1994) Handbook of Wound Dressings. Journal of Wound Care. London: Macmillan Magazines.

Thomas S (1997a) A Prescriber's Guide to Dressings and Wound Management Materials. Value for Money Unit. Welsh Office Health Department.

Thomas S (1997b) A structured approach to the selection of dressings, 14 July (www.worldwidewounds.com/1997/july/Thomas-Guide/Dress-Select).

Thomas S (1998) The use of larval therapy in wound management. Journal of Wound Care 7: 521–524.

Thomas S (2001) An introduction to the use of vacuum assisted closure (www.worldwidewounds.com/2001/may/Thomas/Vacuum-Assisted-Closure.html 09.12.01).

Thomas S, Andrews AM (1999) The effect of hydrogel dressings on maggot development. Journal of Wound Care 8(2): 75–77.

Thomas S, Andrews AM, Hay NP, Bourgoise S (1999) The antimicrobial activity of maggot secretions: results of a preliminary study. Journal of Tissue Viability 9: 127–132.

Thomas S, Andrews AM, Jones M (1998) The use of larval therapy in wound management. Journal of Wound Care 7: 521–524.

Thomas S, Jones M, Shutler S, Jones S (1996) Using larvae in modern wound management. Journal of Wound Care 5(2): 60–69.

Thomas S, Jones M, Wynn K, Fowler T (2001) The current status of maggot therapy in wound healing. British Journal of Nursing Tissue Viability Supplement 10(22): S5–S12.

Thomlinson D (1987) To clean or not to clean. Nursing Times 83(9): 71–75.

Tingle J (1997) Pressure sores: counting the legal cost of nursing neglect. British Journal of Nursing 6: 757–758.

Tong A (1999) Back to basics wound care. Nursing Times Nursing Homes 1(1): 17–19, 21.

Topham J (2000) Sugar for wounds. Journal of Tissue Viability 3: 86–89.

Tortora GJ, Anagnostakos NP (1987) Principles of Anatomy and Physiology, 5th edn. London: Harper & Row.

Touche-Ross Report (1994) The Cost of Pressure Sores. London: Touche Ross.

Turner TD (1982) Which dressing and why? Nursing Times 78(suppl 29): 1–3.

United Kingdom Central Council for Nursing, Midwifery and Health Visiting (1996) Guidelines for Professional Practice. London: UKCC.

United Kingdom Central Council for Nursing, Midwifery and Health Visiting (2004) Guidelines for Records and Record Keeping. London: UKCC.

Value for Money Unit, NHS National Executive (1992) The Nursing Skill Mix in the District Nursing Service. London: HMSO.

Van Rijswijk L (2001) Epidemiology. In: Morison M (ed.), The Prevention and Treatment of Pressure Ulcers. London: Mosby.

Versluysen M (1986) How elderly patients with femoral fractures develop pressure sores in hospital. British Medical Journal 292: 1311–1313.

Vowden KR (1995) Common problems in wound care: wound and ulcer measurement. British Journal of Nursing 4: 775–779.

Vowden KR, Vowden P (1999) Wound debridement, part 1: non-sharp techniques. Journal of Wound Care 8: 237–40.

Wagner FW (1981) The dysvascular foot: a system for diagnosis and treatment. Foot and Ankle 2: 64.

Waldrop J, Doughty D (2000) Wound healing physiology. In: Bryant R (ed.), Acute and Chronic Wounds. Nursing management, 2nd edn. London: Mosby, pp. 17–40.

Wall M (1985) How Wounds Heal. Crewe: The Wellcome Foundation.

Wall P (2001) Promogran Clinical Trial. Johnson & Johnson Advanced Woundcare.

Walsh M, Ford P (1989) Nursing Rituals, Research and Rational Actions. Oxford: Heinemann Nursing.

Walters DP, Gatling W, Mullee MA et al. (1992) The distribution and severity of diabetic foot disease: a community study with comparison to a non-diabetic group. Diabetic Medicine 9: 354–358.

Ward D (2000) Infection control: reducing the psychological effects of isolation. British Journal of Nursing 9: 162–70.

Wardrope J, Smith JA (1992) The Management of Wounds and Burns. Oxford: Oxford University Press.

Warner U, Hall DJ (1986) Pressure sores: a policy for prevention. Nursing Times 82(16): 59–61.

Waterlow J (1985) The Waterlow Card for the prevention and management of pressure sores. Nursing Times 81(48): 49–55.

Waterlow J (1988) Prevention is cheaper than cure. Nursing Times 83(25): 69–70.

Watkins C (2000) Pressure sores. In: Liverpool University Handbook of Geriatric Medicine (www.liv.ac.uk/GeriatricMedicine/cpoa27.htm last accessed July 2003).

Watkins PJ (2003) The diabetic foot. ABC of Diabetes. British Medical Journal 326: 977–979.

Watkins PJ, Drury PL, Howell SL (1997) Diabetes and its Management. Oxford: Blackwell Scientific Publications, pp. 218–238.

Watret L, White R (2001) Surgical wound management: the role of dressings. Nursing Standard 15(44): 59–69.

Weller BF (ed.) (2000) Baillière's Nurses Dictionary, 23rd edn. London: Baillière Tindall.

West JM, Gimbel ML (2000) Acute surgical and traumatic healing In: Bryant R (ed.), Acute and Chronic Wounds, 2nd edn. London: Mosby, pp. 189–196.

Westaby S (1985) Wound Care. London: William Heinemann Medical Books Ltd.

Westaby S, White S (1985) In: Westaby S (ed.), Wound Care. London: William Heinemann Medical Books Ltd, pp. 70–83.

White R (2001) An historical overview of the use of silver in wound management. British Journal of Nursing 10(15): 3–8.

White MI, Jenkinson M, Lloyd DH (1987) The effect of washing on the thickness of the stratum corneum in normal and atopic individuals. British Journal of Dermatology 116: 525.

Wiersema-Bryant LA, Kraemer BA (2000) Vascular and neuropathic wounds: the diabetic wound. In: Bryant RA (ed.), Acute and Chronic Wounds. Nursing management, 2nd edn. London: Mosby, pp. 301–315.

Willcock J, Hughes J, Tickle S, Rossiter G, Johnson C, Pye H (2000) Pressure sores in children – the acute hospital perspective. Journal of Tissue Viability 11: 139–142.

Williams S, Watret L, Pell J (2001) Case-mix adjusted incidence of pressure ulcers in acute medical and surgical wards. Journal of Tissue Viability 11: 139–142.

Wilson J (1995) Infection Control in Clinical Practice. London: Baillière Tindall.

Wilson J (1999) Clinical governance and the potential implications for tissue viability. Journal of Tissue Viability 9(3): 95–98.

Winter GD (1962) Formation of the scab and the rate of epithelialisation of superficial wounds in the skin of the domestic pig. Nature 193: 293–294.

Working Party Report (1998) Revised guidelines for the control of methicillin resistant Staphylococcus aureus infection in hospitals. Journal of Hospital Infection 39: 253–290.

World Health Organization (2003) Diabetes estimates and projections (www.who.int/ncd/dia/databases4.htm, last accessed 28 December 2003).

Wysocki AB (1992) Skin. In: Bryant RA (ed.), Acute and Chronic Wounds. Nursing management. St Louis, MO: Mosby Year Book, pp. 1–30.

Wysocki AB (2000) Anatomy and physiology of skin and soft tissue. In: Bryant R (ed.), Acute and Chronic Wounds. Nursing management, 2nd edn. London: Mosby, pp. 1–16.

Xakellis GC (1993) Guidelines for the prediction and prevention of pressure ulcers. Journal of the American Board of Family Practitioners 6: 269–278.

Young T (1995) Common problems in wound care: overgranulation. British Journal of Nursing 4: 169–170.

Young JB, Dobrzanski S (1992) Pressure sores: epidemiology and current management concepts. Drugs and Aging 2: 42–57.

Index

237